OPTIMAL HEALTH SERIES

ZZZ's

Optimal Sleep, Optimal Health

**How to Overcome Your Insomnia
And Sleep Disorders Naturally**

Bob Armstrong

Independently Self-Published
First Edition

ISBN-13: 978-1719360296
ISBN-10: 1719360294

Ultimate Health Series
Modesto, California

DISCLAIMER

All attempts have been made to verify the information in this book; however, neither the author, nor the publisher assumes any responsibility for errors, omissions, or contrary interpretations of the content within. Neither the author nor the publisher assumes any responsibility or liability on behalf of the purchaser or reader of this book.

This book is for entertainment purposes only, and so the views and opinions of the author should not be taken as expert instruction or commands. The reader is responsible for his or her actions.

It's always recommend that you seek to obtain medical advice from licensed physicians for medical questions. This book is not intended to offer professional advice as a substitute for good medical information provided by your medical team.

Thank you.

Buyer Bonus Material

As of a way of thanking you for your purchase I've included a bonus report at the **end of this book**. I hope you enjoy this. Thank you.

Other Books to Check Out

As part of the **Optimal Health Series** please pickup your copy of these books from <u>Bob Armstrong</u> too. Thank you!

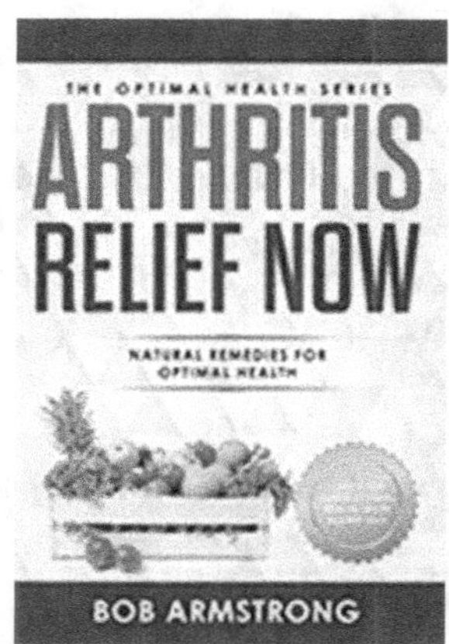

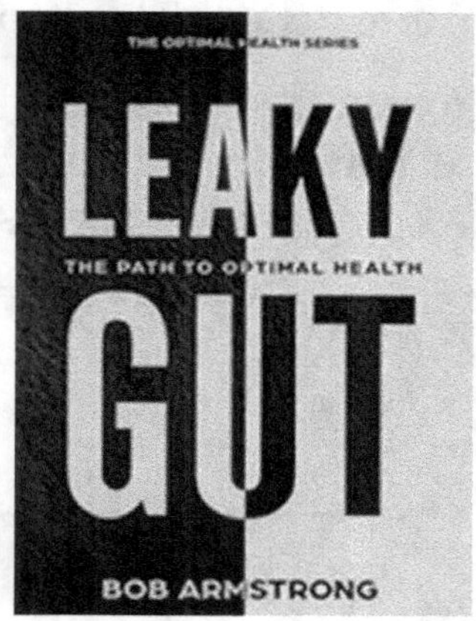

<u>Other Books Slated To Come Out Soon:</u>

Quit Smoking Now!

DEDICATION

Special thanks and dedication to my eternal companion, Denise who's support and love are unmatched. This book was written for her.

Also to you who has struggled with sleepless nights for far too long. May this aid you in your quest for a good night's sleep!

Sweet Dreams!

Contents

INTRODUCTION

"I love sleep. My life has the tendency to fall apart when I'm awake, you know?" ~ Ernest Hemingway

"I just want a good night's sleep." Ever said that before? Oh yeah. All of us have said that, at one time or another. Some people I've met and spoken to over the years have made that comment their daily mantra though and that's a major concern.

Not everyone views sleep in the same way. For some people it's the most pleasurable time of the day, and still others would rather do without it altogether. Trials and tribulations are an undeniable part of our life experience. Some people value sleep as a nourishing gap in their existence. A time where they can lie down in a comfortable bed and disengage from the world during those few hours. Some value sleep for its regenerative properties. You can go to sleep after a physically and mentally hard day's work and awake refreshed, physically healed, and with new perspective.

And yet still others see sleep as a distraction. Something they have to "go through" to prevent total fatigue and burnout. Not pleasurable at all.

As you read this book, I want you to think of sleep as a basic foundational process your body needs that can have an amazing transformational effect on you.

There are at least three health pillars in life to consider for optimal health and living. Sleep, nutrition and exercise. While you and only you can control what you eat, which supplements you take and your daily exercise regimen, sleep may be the most important pillar of all and sometimes a little more difficult to control. Did you know that a lot goes on in your body while you sleep? While you sleep, cellular repair and growth is happening, blood pressure drops, breathing slows down, blood flow moves to the muscles, and tissues are repaired, according to the National Sleep Foundation. Hormones, such as the human growth hormones, are secreted at this time as well. Your body is recharging and regenerating.

How do you overcome sleep issues? There's no single, easy answer, of course, but it makes perfect sense to implement a lifestyle approach first that makes a difference. That's what this book is about. Dr. Mehmet Oz has said, "Sleep on a schedule. Deep sleep is the most important sleep; it promotes muscle mass by generating growth hormone. Turn off the computer and the TV well before bed time, so your brain releases melatonin." Lifestyle changes can be small twists in our daily routines but they can make significant changes in overall sleep wellness.

I've discovered that this lifestyle approach is really a recognition of things we generally innately know, but aren't doing and need to be reminded of. For example, sometimes we know that we can overcome our sleeplessness and insomnia with a little better planning, better food selection throughout our day, recognizing technology interference and how it can physically change how our minds react, and stress and how we react to the pressures of the day. These, and others, then become the causes of insomnia. Now we know that doing something about insomnia becomes our challenge. So let's jump in.

Sleep serves both a physical, emotional and psychological need that is required throughout your life. You know that sleep is important, and that you don't feel well when you don't get it. Unfortunately, in our fast-paced, modern world filled with distractions, work, family demands, stress and technology, sleep is often the first thing we sacrifice.

After all, we all only get 24 hours each day. Why not try to fit as many things as possible into these 24 hours? Right? Perhaps you have an important project that's due tomorrow. Well, you can always cut out a couple of hours of sleep to get it done, right?

Unfortunately, that is how more and more of us are viewing sleep. We see it as an annoyance or an interruption to getting more things done in a day. Teenagers and adults are all suffering the negative consequences of this attitude towards sleep. Health suffers when sleep is put on the back burner. (More on this later.)

High-quality sleep is just as important for overall health as eating well and exercising regularly. Nevertheless, many people seem to have trouble falling asleep, wake up frequently or fail to wake up feeling fully rested. This makes it challenging to maintain optimal health and well-being.

There are some people who are trying to prioritize their sleep, and that's good. They really want to get more sleep or want to sleep better, but they continue to wake up feeling unrefreshed. Perhaps, the stress in their lives is interfering with their sleep, or there are things that they need to change to get the sleep their bodies crave?

In any case, it is time to see sleep for what it really is, "a necessary component to good health, both in the short-term and the long term." Getting adequate, quality sleep is just as important as what you eat and how much you exercise. Not getting enough sleep is linked to numerous health concerns and diseases. Even serious diseases, such as cancer, have been linked to inadequate levels of sleep and disrupted sleep systems in people who work late shifts.

The main focus of this book is to help you understand the stages of and purpose for sleep, the importance of sleep for your health, and some ways to start improving your sleep. The truth is that you may not realize that sleep plays an even more important role in your health than just keeping you from being tired. Once you understand this, you will never again underscore the importance of sleep for your health.

ONE

Understanding the Different Stages of Sleep

"I love to sleep. I'd sleep all day if I could." ~ Miley Cyrus

How big a problem is sleep deprivation and insomnia? Did you know that 50 to 70 million Americans are affected by chronic sleep disorders and intermittent sleep problems that can significantly diminish health, alertness and safety? True. Untreated sleep disorders have been linked to hypertension, heart disease, stroke, depression, diabetes and other chronic diseases. Sleep problems can take many forms and can involve too little sleep, too much sleep or inadequate quality of sleep.

The Institute of Medicine recently estimated in its report, *Sleep Disorders and Sleep Deprivation: An Unmet Public Health Problem,* that "hundreds of billions of dollars a year are spent on direct medical costs related to sleep disorders such as doctor visits, hospital services, prescriptions, and over-the-counter medications." Sleep problems and lack of sleep can affect everything from personal and work productivity to behavioral and relationship problems. Sleep problems can have serious consequences. According to the National Highway Traffic Safety Administration, drowsy driving claims more than 1,500 lives and causes at least 100,000 motor vehicle crashes each year.

Compounding the problem is the fact that most people know when to seek medical help for physical discomfort such as fever or pain—but sleep problems are often overlooked or even ignored. In fact, the overwhelming majority of people with sleep disorders are undiagnosed and untreated. Source: https://sleepfoundation.org.

Sleep shouldn't be a luxury, but rather an absolute necessity! It allows your brain and body to recover after periods of wakefulness. Specifically, sleep restores your body's ability to function, to repair body tissues, create hormones, consolidate memories and learning, and regulate mood. Sleep makes up such an important part of our lives, that there are people who spend the majority of their careers dedicated to the topic.

Whether you experience an occasional day of sleepiness, or you feel like you spend most of your days in a sleep-deprived state, it is important to understand the different stages of sleep. This can then help you improve the quality of your sleep so that you will enhance your functioning when you are awake.

No one stage of sleep is more important than another. Studies have shown that each stage plays a distinctive role in your health. In addition, your sleep follows a predictable pattern every night. In other words, actual stages exist where your brain waves change, the ability to be awakened easily changes, and there are specific times when you experience vivid dreaming.

Sleep can be divided into two major categories-

REM sleep and **non-REM** sleep.

REM stands for "Rapid Eye Movement."

First, we will discuss **non-REM sleep**, as this is always the starting point for healthy adults when you fall asleep. According to the National Sleep Foundation, three phases of non-REM sleep exist, each lasting from 5 to 15 minutes, and making up about 75% of your sleep at night. You must pass through all three phases before you reach the REM phase about 90 minutes after you first fall asleep. This cycle of non-REM – REM sleep repeats itself throughout the night, with the first full cycle lasting between 70 and 100 minutes. The second and later sleep cycles last between 90 and 120 minutes.

The three phases of non-REM sleep include:

N1 (also known as Stage 1):

Your eyes are closed, and you feel drowsy. Your brain activity starts to slow down. This is the transition period from wakefulness to sleep. During this time, you may experience the sensation of falling, as well as a muscle jerk that wakes you up. This is normal. Muscle tone continues to be high.

In this stage, you are still easily awakened, and you will not feel too drowsy or disoriented if woken up. If awakened from this stage, you may not even be aware that you had fallen asleep. This stage usually lasts no more than seven minutes.

N2 (also known as Stage 2):

Your brain waves become even slower, but they have occasional bursts of activity. Your body temperature goes down. If you are awakened from this stage, you will know that you have been sleeping.

N3 (also known as Stages 3 and 4):

Recordings of your brain waves at these stages demonstrate slow waves called, "delta waves." Your body temperature decreases even more, your breathing is slower, and your blood pressure decreases. This is what is typically known as the "deep sleep" stage.

It is harder to wake someone up during this stage of sleep, but if you are awakened, you will feel groggy, you may feel disoriented, and it will take some time to feel alert.

This restorative stage of sleep is important for your body to recover from the fatigue it undergoes from the previous hours you were awake, and to build up energy for the next day. Your body also rebuilds bone and muscle, repairs tissues, and increases the functioning of your immune system, during this time of sleep. Growth hormone is also released, which is important for muscle development and growth.

Most of Stages 3 and 4 slow-wave sleep occurs in the early hours of the night. In other words, as the night progresses, you spend less and less of your sleep in N3.

REM sleep

As previously mentioned, **REM stands for "rapid eye movement."** Your heart rate and breathing increase during REM sleep. Your breathing sounds shallow and irregular. Your eyes move rapidly, hence the term, rapid eye movement. Your muscle tone decreases so significantly that it resembles paralysis.

This stage of sleep typically occurs ninety minutes after you first fall asleep, and approximately every ninety minutes thereafter in your sleep that night. The first REM sleep period lasts no more than ten minutes, and continues to increase each cycle of the night, resulting in being around an hour long for the final REM episode of the night. As a result, most of your REM sleep occurs in the early morning hours. Although dreaming occurs at all stages of sleep, you have the most vivid dreams during REM sleep when the brain is quite active.

You move through all of these stages in a sequential manner, repeating the stages as you sleep.

TWO

How Much Sleep Do You Need?

"The amount of sleep required by the average person is five minutes more." ~ Wilson Mizener

Considering that we spend one third of our lives asleep, knowing how much sleep is required is a good question. However, it often comes with an over-generalization.

For example, in March 2015, the National Sleep Foundation came up with some guidelines on how much sleep that people, of different ages, should be getting.

The recommendations were for healthy people with normal sleep patterns. The appropriate duration of sleep for a newborn, for example, is 14 – 17 hours. Whereas, teenagers are reported to be fine with 8 – 10 hours. Young adults and middle-age adults should be aiming for 7 – 9 hours per night, and older adults should try to get 7 – 8 hours of sleep. So although the duration of sleep varies by age, there is a similarity amongst age groups.

The truth is that sleep is complex and multifactorial. The "magic" number of sleep that you have probably heard the most is "eight hours." Although the National Sleep Foundation came out with these guidelines, some people who work in the field still advocate a more common-sense approach to determining how much sleep you need. This will be discussed in what follows.

If you asked a stranger how much sleep you require, he would probably tell you "eight hours." However, the fact is that this stranger knows nothing about you about your lifestyle, your job, and your stresses. It would be like you trying to determine how many calories the stranger across the street should be consuming every day without you knowing if she exercises, if she is muscle building, or if she is pregnant.

With that in mind, it makes more sense to monitor how you feel, and determine what sleep duration is best for you. You can monitor things like:

How long it takes you to fall asleep – If you fall asleep as soon as your head hits the pillow, then you may need more sleep than others. If it takes you a long time to fall asleep, then perhaps you are sleeping too much or are distracted at bedtime.

Does your body wake up before your alarm? – Your body knows when it is time to wake up. Your internal clock is much wiser than any alarm clock, that you buy, will ever be.

How do you feel during the day? – If you are struggling to keep your eyes open, then you may need more sleep. If you are able to stay awake and alert, then the amount of sleep you got is probably fine.

By monitoring these things, it can help you adjust your schedule accordingly, and get the desired amount of sleep that you need.

THREE

Why is Sleep so Important for Your Health?

"Sleep is the golden chain that ties health and our bodies together." ~ Thomas Dekker

You already know that sleep is important. Without adequate amounts, you feel sleepy. You may also experience other obvious signs and symptoms such as crankiness, headaches, and/or trouble concentrating. However, there are even more serious consequences of not getting enough shut-eye. These are explained in what follows:

Your Physical Health –

1. Increased Risk of Obesity due to the following factors –

    a.) No energy

If you do not get adequate sleep at night, you may delay getting out of bed in the morning, because you are too sleepy. As a result, now you do not have enough time to make a healthy breakfast and pack a healthy lunch. You rush out of the house, and you pick up a coffee and donut on the way to work. If you packed a lunch, you eat whatever you threw together at the last minute in the morning, or you buy whatever is on the menu at the cafeteria that day. On your way home, you are tired and you do not feel like spending an hour in the kitchen preparing something, so you decide to get take-out pizza. You decide to skip the gym that night, because you are just too tired.

You can see how this becomes a vicious cycle and can result in weight gain.

b.) Your body's use of glucose is impaired

Normally, when you eat, your body's cells are supposed to use the energy (glucose). However, when you are sleep deprived, your body is not as efficient at doing this. This makes you feel more tired, hungrier so you eat more, and it also increases your chance of diabetes.

c.) Your hormones are thrown out-of-whack.

A hormone called, cortisol, is produced by your adrenal glands. It is commonly referred to as one of the "stress hormones." Cortisol increases with lack of sleep, and it also makes it harder to sleep. Normally, your cortisol levels should be highest in the morning so that it is easy to wake up, and lowest in the evenings when your body prepares for sleep and as it sleeps. High levels of cortisol, when it should be low in your body, is linked to weight gain, obesity, and diabetes.

A couple other important hormones that are affected by lack of sleep include ghrelin and leptin. Ghrelin is the hormone that tells you when you are hungry, and when it's time to eat.

In contrast, leptin is a hormone that tells you when you are full, and that it is time to stop eating. Unfortunately, when you don't get enough sleep, ghrelin increases and leptin decreases, putting you at risk of weight gain.

2. **Increased Risk of Diseases** – As already mentioned above, lack of sleep increases potential for weight gain and unstable blood sugars, which then increases your risk of diabetes.

Heart disease is also higher if you are chronically sleep deprived. According to the National Sleep Foundation, despite exercise, age, weight, and smoking habits, your risk of heart disease goes up if you do not get enough sleep. Although the exact causes are not known, lack of sleep is linked to high blood pressure, high cholesterol, and increased inflammation in the body. All sleep-deprived individuals are at risk of this, but people with sleep apnea tend to have even higher rates of heart disease than those without the medical problem.

3. **Lowered Immune System Functioning –** Your immune system is what protects your body from germs. When your body encounters germs, your body goes to work to fight off the invaders. However, when you don't get enough sleep, your immune system does not function as well, increasing your susceptibility to colds, flu, and other ailments. The simple explanation is that your immune system cannot produce the germ-fighting cells that it needs when you aren't getting enough sleep. Your body is effective at restoring these fighter cells when you sleep.

4. **Your Sex Life Suffers –** This actually could have been included in the topic of hormone disruption above. This is because the sex hormone, testosterone, is reduced in men and women who are leading sleep-deprived lives. This, in turn, results in a decreased interest in sex for both genders, erectile dysfunction in males, and reduced vaginal lubrication in females.

5. Increased Risk of Injuries and Accidents – When you are tired, your concentration and focus is poor. Therefore, this puts you at increased risk of workplace injuries and car accidents.

Your Cognitive, Mental, & Emotional Health

Pulling all-nighters is not only a bad idea for your physical health, it also negatively impacts your mental, cognitive, and emotional health. More people are recognizing that the days of bragging about being able to function with only a few hours of sleep, is really a health hazard and not something with which to mess around.

Here are 7 ways that sleep deprivation affects these areas of your health:

1. **Decreased Ability to Handle Stress** – Stressful situations are difficult enough to handle when you have gotten a good sleep. When you get less than ideal amounts of sleep, and you are dealing with stress, your ability to do this well, deteriorates significantly. You may get angry, yell, cry, or do things that you normally wouldn't do if you had gotten a good night of sleep.

2. **Altered Mood** – This one seems obvious. You already know that you feel irritable and short-tempered when you don't get enough sleep. Chronic lack of sleep, however, also increases your chances of depression and anxiety.

3. **Decreased Ability to Think & Learn** – Your ability to concentrate and focus on tasks, make decisions, and carry through with them, is hampered a great deal with lack of sleep.

In addition, your ability to learn new things is also reduced. Sleep is known to help with new learning, and it is probably the reason why babies and young children sleep so much as they are constantly learning and adapting to their environments. New learning does not end with childhood, so adequate sleep continues to play an important role in adults. In addition, your brain assimilates information as you sleep, helping you to retain information.

4. **Negatively Impacts Relationships** – Because of your reduced ability to handle stress and your increased irritability, it makes sense that your personal and work relationships will suffer. This may also take a toll on your self-esteem as friendships and relationships are ruined, and you find that you have no one with which to talk.

5. **Reduced Judgment Skills** – Although this also falls under the inability to think, it deserves its own bullet point. If your judgment and insight is lacking due to poor sleep, your

decision-making skills will be affected. You may make more impulsive decisions, or do things that are potentially unsafe while driving, for example. Your ability to assess situations accurately decreases.

6. **Poor Memory** – Again, this goes back to the inability to concentrate and focus on what is happening around you. If you do not register things in your short-term memory, it is impossible for the brain to convert memories to long term ones.

7. **Slowed Reaction Time** – Sleepiness when driving, has been described as being as dangerous as driving under the influence of alcohol. If you mix lack of sleep and alcohol, it makes you even more dangerous behind the wheel.

Not only is driving dangerous when you lack sleep, working in certain industries or professions, when sleep-deprived, can be extremely dangerous to you and others. For example, construction workers, truck drivers and police officers are a few of the many professions that require alertness and the ability to react quickly.

FOUR

5 Ways to Make Sleep a Priority

The woods are lovely, dark and deep. But I have promises to keep, and miles to go before I sleep.~ Robert Frost

Hopefully, the importance of sleep and how it impacts your physical and mental well-being is becoming clear. With that being said, you need to make sleep a priority in your life. Think about how much better you'll feel, and what you can accomplish if you work on improving your sleep.

If your sleep does not improve, no matter what you try, you should speak to your doctor as there could be underlying medical or psychological problems.

Here are some tips on how to learn to prioritize your sleep, and how to get to bed at a reasonable hour:

1. **Establish a bedtime routine** – Just as children benefit from routines, so do adults. It is beneficial to create a routine where you start getting ready at least an hour before lights go out. This may include having a bath or shower (not too hot though as this could impede falling asleep easily), getting into your pajamas, having a light snack, meditation, prayer or reading a book. Set your bedtime. I've always appreciated the fact that if I needed 7 hours of sleep and wanted to be up early, say 5am, then I just worked it backwards and went to bed at 10pm. Remember, "early to bed, early to rise makes a man healthy, wealthy and wise. (Ben Franklin).

2. **Set up a pleasant atmosphere** – You want to set up your bedroom so that it is cozy, and so that you enjoy retreating to it at the end of a busy day. Pay attention to the colors of your walls. Choose calming, soothing paint colors such as soft grays, lavender, or sage. Set up a lamp with a soft yellow or red light. Avoid lights that emit blue wave lengths. Decorate your walls in such a way that it adds to the beauty of the room.

3. **Recognize the difference between being busy and being productive** – Have you ever found yourself wasting time at the end of the day, because you are tired, but it feels like it is too early to go to bed? For example, you might be surfing the internet or checking your emails for the 20th time that day, but you aren't doing anything productive. Instead, you are just keeping yourself busy. Learn to recognize when you are doing this, so that you can spend your time more wisely, and you don't steal time from your bedtime routine.

4. **Remind yourself of this saying, "Rome wasn't built in a day."** - When you look around your house at the end of the day, you can always find something else to do before you head off to bed – dirty dishes in the sink, crumbs on the floor that need to be swept, or another email waiting to be answered. This is never going to change. Realize that there will always be things that don't get done in a day, and that you can start fresh the next day after a good night of sleep.

5. **Avoid emotional and financial conversations before bedtime** – Evenings are not a good time to be having difficult conversations with friends or family. Talking about your financial situation, such as your outstanding credit card balance, should also not be done before bedtime. Instead, these conversations, including texts and emails, should be reserved for daytime when you have the energy, and when they are not going to cause you extra stress right before it is time to fall asleep.

Seeking out a medical professional to conduct a sleep study with you is another approach that should be considered as well. Depending on your insurance plan and other factors, your primary care physician may start your evaluation by running some tests for specific medical disorders that are known to affect sleep.

Your physician might even be able to diagnose a sleep problem based solely on your symptoms and recommend initial treatments. At some point, you may be referred to a sleep specialist for a more extensive assessment of your sleep complaints and for more specific treatments.

If this occurs, be sure to ask your physician to refer you to a certified sleep physician. Certification requires that a physician undergo formal training and pass an examination in sleep disorders to demonstrate a higher level of expertise. To check if your sleep physician is certified, or to find a sleep professional, go to www.absm.org. This may be a good step for some patients with chronic conditions.

FIVE

7 Tips to Improve Your Sleep Tonight

"At the end of the day, sleep is a barometer of your emotional health. And so if you're not in the right place where you need to be, then you're going to have voices keeping you up at night because you have to work through those issues."
~ Dr. Mehmet Oz

Sleep hygiene involves doing a number of different things that prepare your body for sleep, and allow it to have quality sleep so that you can be alert the next day. Following a regular bedtime routine is one aspect of sleep hygiene, but there are many other things that you can do to improve your sleep starting now. These include:

1. **Caffeine cut-off times** – You know that caffeine should be limited before bedtime, but when exactly in the day should you stop drinking caffeinated beverages? It is probably earlier than you realize. A general guideline is no later than 2 p.m. This is

because studies have shown that consumption of caffeine even six hours before bedtime, can cause disturbances in sleep quality. Although you may not notice the effects of the caffeine when you go to sleep, your body's sleep quality will still be poorer.

Therefore, recommendations include drinking caffeinated beverages in the morning hours, and very early afternoon. Drink no more than 400 mg of caffeine per day, which is equal to about 4 cups of coffee. Any more than that, and you should be choosing decaffeinated coffee or tea. And don't forget that caffeine is also found in cola, hot chocolate, cocoa, and some over-the-counter and prescription pain medications.

2. **Limit alcohol intake** – Although alcohol is a central nervous system depressant, and causes you to feel sleepy, it actually disrupts your sleep quality. Your body does not enter the deeper sleep cycle, which is necessary to restore your energy for the next day. In addition, as the alcohol wears off, your brain "reboots" causing disruption in the normal brain wave pattern that allows for quality sleep.

3. **Go to bed at the same time every night – give or take 20 minutes.** You have probably heard this advice before. By doing so, you can actually train your body to wake up without an alarm clock. Work your "must be up in the morning time" backwards with the appropriate sleep needed. If 5am is your regular wake-up time, and 7 hours is what you need for a complete rest, then you're in bed no later than 10pm.

4. **Have sex before sleep time** – Sleep hygiene experts tell you to reserve your bed only for sleep and sex. However, let's take it a step further. Studies show that sex, in conjunction with orgasms, is a great way to end the day before you nod off. This is because sex can distract you (be sure to put away your phone and other electronic devices!), and it promotes the release of "feel good" hormones that relax you and reduce your perception of pain.

5. **Set up your bedroom environment** – In addition to setting up a pleasant setting that is cozy

and has calming colors, you need to limit the light in your bedroom before you fall asleep and during sleep. Even the light from your alarm clock can negatively affect your sleep, so cover the light emitting from it. In addition, be sure to use room-darkening shades over the windows. Keep the room quiet. If you live on a busy, loud street, for example, you may need to create white noise using a fan, or you can use a phone app. Just be sure that, if it is a fan that it is not blowing directly on you. Keep your bedroom temperature lower, as this will promote better, deeper sleep.

6. **Get up after 20 minutes in bed, if you haven't fallen asleep yet** – There is no point to staying in bed tossing and turning. All it does it frustrate you, which impedes the goal – falling asleep. Instead, it is better to get up and do something quiet. The goal remains the same. You want to get back to bed and get some sleep. Try taking your mind off the issue by reading a book (not a tablet or smartphone as the blue light emitted will increase your wakefulness),

meditating, listening to calming music, or doing some relaxation exercises.

7. Use sleep tools to help you fall asleep faster —

"<u>Prevention</u>" magazine, states that the number one reason why people find themselves having trouble getting to sleep is due to a busy mind that just won't seem to shut down. Other reasons include stress, illness, travel, or other interruptions to your normal everyday routine. Here are some tools that can help you get to sleep easier. **For example:**

- Sleep mask to block out light
- **Sleep-aid and nap machine** products may also produce other soothing **sounds**, such as music, rain, wind, highway traffic and ocean waves mixed with—or modulated by—**white noise. White noise** generators **are** often used by people with tinnitus to mask their symptoms.

- **Blackout shades** helps prepare your body and brain for sleep.

- **Getting earplugs** like **these** that mold to your ears is an inexpensive and effective way to block out noise.

- **Sleep Friendly Blue-light bulbs.**

- **Smart device phone apps** have a Bluetooth breathing sensor. The device uses guided breathing techniques to help the user fall asleep.

- **Essential Oil Diffuser.** Essential oils are very popular these days for a variety of uses, including inducing natural sleep.

- **Your routine which includes:**

1. Warm bath

2. Light stretching and exercising

3. Writing in your journal

4. Deep breathing exercises

5. A cup of caffeine-free herbal tea 30 minutes before bed

- **Wear socks**. People who tend to have cold extremities may find it hard to sleep if their feet start to get cold in the middle of the night. Wrap them up with some warm socks before bed to prevent this. It's surprising how this can really make a difference.

SIX

What Does Your Biological Clock Have to Do With Your Sleep?

"Without enough sleep, we all become tall two-year-olds." ~JoJo Jensen, Dirt Farmer Wisdom, 2002

We all have a biological clock. This biological clock is sometimes referred to as your **circadian rhythm**, or your sleep-wake cycle. In fact, there is a small "part" in your brain that controls all of this. It controls when your brain and other organs secrete chemical messengers, known as hormones to other parts of your body to cause things to happen in your body. Even when this part is removed from the brain, it continues to function all on its own!

The reason that it is important to have a general understanding of how this biological clock works, is so that you can understand HOW to improve and program your sleep. If you understand some of the hormones involved, for example, it will help you know whether you should be using particular natural supplements to help your sleep. In what follows, you will learn more about two specific hormones (melatonin and cortisol) and a compound (adenosine) that are important for your sleep and how they play an important role in the functioning of your biological clock.

Melatonin

Melatonin is a hormone that is produced in your brain. It is actually synthesized from another hormone in your brain called serotonin. Melatonin production is stimulated by darkness, or when blue light is no longer entering your eyes. It is one hormone that contributes to feeling sleepy. It is also known to play a role in the reduction of aging in your brain and body, as well as to have cancer-fighting properties.

Melatonin production comes to a halt when blue light enters your eyes by way of daylight. When your brain sense blue light, melatonin production stops. As an aside, these blue wave lengths are what make the sky look blue when it scatters in the atmosphere. It is also important to note that special "daylight lamps", used by people with **Seasonal Affective Disorder (SAD)** or the "winter blues", also provide the eyes with blue light required to elevate mood and reduce the fatigue associated with this disorder.

As you can see, blue light is what regulates your wake and sleep cycles. Blue light is emitted by natural sources such as the sun, but also by artificial sources like electronic devices, such as televisions, computers, smartphones, as well as most household and workplace lights.

It is therefore important to reduce blue light exposure in the evenings and while you sleep, in order to get a quality sleep. Our bodies were never designed to need blue light at nighttime, but the use of artificial light sources has made it difficult to avoid. Your body continues to think that it is daytime, and does not produce adequate volumes of melatonin, thus confusing your body's natural cycles. This is a modern-day issue, because years ago, lanterns and oil lamps were the norm and these items did not emit blue light. That is why you have some of your best sleeps when camping, as long as you pay attention not to use artificial lighting in the evenings. The setting sun and the natural light of the fire do not interfere with your body's biological clock, and actually encourage it to do what it's supposed to do – release melatonin required for sleep.

Cortisol

Another important hormone is Cortisol. It affects your sleep. Under normal, healthy conditions, cortisol levels should rise in the mornings, and decrease in the evenings. In contrast, the sleep hormone, melatonin, is supposed to rise in the evenings when darkness prevails, and decrease in the mornings for waking. So as melatonin levels decrease, your cortisol levels pick up. Both hormones are similar though, in that they both work on an approximate 24-hour cycle in your body, supporting your body's biological clock.

Cortisol is known as one of the "fight or flight stress hormones." It is released by your adrenal glands in your body. When released, cortisol increases your blood sugar levels, so that your muscles and brain get the energy needed to act. It helps wake you up, and keeps you alert during the daytime. It is typically highest at 8 a.m., and lowest between the hours of midnight and 4 a.m.

But too much cortisol is not a good thing either, especially when your cortisol levels remain high throughout the evening. This occurs when you are experiencing emotional or physical (i.e. sickness) stress. Even having an upsetting conversation, learning of exciting news, or watching a thrilling television show in the evening, can increase your cortisol levels. These elevated cortisol levels in the evenings can then keep you from falling asleep and prevent you from having a restful sleep.

Unfortunately, if your adrenal glands continue to secrete cortisol, as is the case during periods of prolonged stress, eventually they burn out (this is what is referred to as "adrenal fatigue"), and normal surges of cortisol in the morning no longer occur. In fact, if your adrenal glands are no longer producing adequate volumes of cortisol, your blood sugars levels are not going to be high enough at nighttime, so your sleep will suffer as you wake up earlier from the brain signaling its hunger. To complicate matters, if you do not get enough sleep one night, your cortisol levels will be elevated the next night.

As you can see, your body's systems and hormones are all inter-related. What happens to one, affects another, and together, they impact the quality and quantity of your sleep.

Adenosine

This is another chemical naturally found in your body. Without getting into the complex chemistry, all you need to know is that adenosine builds up each hour that you are awake causing you to become sleepy. Adenosine is in every cell in your body and is a by-product of your cells working and using energy in your body. It works in conjunction with melatonin, which is released in response to darkness. Adenosine breaks down when you sleep.

It is believed that when you exert more energy through physical exercise and physical labor, that your adenosine levels build up more, causing you to feel sleepier at nighttime. That is why you notice feeling very sleepy after a long day of skiing or surfing, for example, compared to when you exert less energy during the day.

A vigorous gym workout can work the same way too. But beware of your own body. Some folks react exactly the opposite and find it hard to nod off.

SEVEN

7 Ways to Avoid Blue Light at Night

"Nothing cures insomnia like the realization that it's time to get up." ~ Author Unknown

Perhaps you are doing your best to take care of your body - eating healthy foods, getting regular exercise, and reducing your stress levels. Sleep is also part of a healthy lifestyle – both quantity and quality. Studies, however, show that people are sleeping less. One of the reasons for this is the exposure to blue light at the wrong time of day.

Blue light is found in the sun (as well as other color wave lengths). Blue light has a shorter wave length, and it is energizing and mood enhancing. When this light hits your eyes in the mornings, it sends signals to your brain telling you that it is time to wake up. This is controlled by melatonin production being turned off.

Whereas, when the sun sets, you are not exposed to its blue light until sunrise again.

Unfortunately, you continue to be exposed to blue light even after the sun sets. This is because of artificial lighting and technology (TV's, computers, tablets, etc.) in your home. The invention of the light bulb and other technology has tricked your brain into thinking that it is still daytime. It results in increasing your evening alertness, as well as changing your body's biological clock (also referred to as the circadian rhythm) and hormones so that sleep is delayed. In fact, any artificial light exposure in the evening is an issue. Even dim lamps can emit enough blue light to disrupt your sleep rhythms!

Obviously, it is difficult to survive in today's world in total evening darkness. You could read by candlelight, but that is probably not possible when you have worked all day and have evening responsibilities with your children, for example.

So what steps can you take to avoid or reduce blue light exposure in the evening?

1. **Avoid the use of technology at least two hours before bedtime.** This means not using your computer, tablet, smartphone, and television, for example. These items all emit blue light, and prevent the production of melatonin, the latter which is needed to cause you to become sleepy.

2. **If you absolutely have to use technology or to be in bright light in the evening, use <u>blue-blocking glasses</u>.** These can also be useful for evening and nightshift workers. Be sure you buy them from a good source. Your optometrist may be an invaluable resource to make specific recommendations. You can also find them sold online through various outlets. The various glasses above are from Amazon.

3. **Maximize exposure to light during the day.** This does not mean sit in the sun all day, otherwise you will potentially end up with other serious problems such as skin cancer or damage to your eyes (cataracts and age-related macular degeneration are accelerated by too much blue light

exposure). Instead, it appears that maximum daytime exposure results in lessening the effects of being exposed to light at night. Plan to take a walk outdoors over your lunch break at the same time every day. This same-day exposure to sunlight can aid your body's internal clock.

In winter, or if you spend days at work with no exposure to natural light, be sure to use a light box that provides you with plenty of blue light. You can use it before you go to work, while you are eating your breakfast or applying your cosmetics, for example. If you sit at a desk, you can use a light box at work.

4. **You can adjust the colors of your screens on your smartphones, computers, and tablets to warmer, shorter wave lengths.** Set it up so that it happens automatically every evening, and results in little to no exposure to blue light at this time.

5. **Choose light bulbs that emit less or no blue light**, and emit more reddish or warmer hues. <u>**See various bulbs here**</u>.

6. **During sleep, cover any lights on your alarm clock or other devices at night.** Use room-darkening shades to avoid exposure from streetlights or your neighbor's lights. Wear a sleep mask.

7. **Go camping** – Whether you like camping or not, this is one of the best ways to avoid blue light exposure at night. It is also a great way to reset your body's biological clock. Therefore, you may want to rethink your family vacation this year. If you are looking for a restful vacation, camping may be the best way to go about getting that.

EIGHT

Recommendations for Artificial Lighting for Quality Sleep – Say What?

"It is a common experience that a problem difficult at night is resolved in the morning after the committee of sleep has worked on it." ~ John Steinbeck

Artificial lighting is a norm in modern-day society. When the sun sets, the lights also go on in homes and businesses across the world. Even though studies are demonstrating the importance of limiting exposure to light (blue, in particular) before bedtime, it is highly unlikely that people are going to adopt "lightless" evenings or start using oil lamps or candles again.

Even NASA recognized that the fluorescent lighting on the International Space Station, was disrupting the sleep of astronauts. NASA has since changed the bulbs to ones that do not emit blue light all night.

This begs another question. If you are going to be exposed to light in the evenings, what should you know about light bulbs in order to make better choices that have a less-negative impact on your sleep?

Red light bulbs – You know that blue light disrupts your hormones and sleep levels. Red light, on the other hand, is conducive to good sleep. These are the best lights to use in your bedroom, and for reading a paper book. Red nightlights are also available, if you need to use one in a sleeping area. You can buy them online, at Amazon, for example.

Incandescent light bulbs – These are the type of bulbs that Thomas Edison brought to the marketplace. Until recent years, these were the most popular bulbs used in homes across North America. Some countries no longer use them, mostly because they are less energy efficient. They also do not last as long – around 1000 hours - as other types created in more recent years. However, they do produce warmer hues, and although not as good as red light bulbs, they are an option for cutting down on blue light. Keep reading for other options though.

Compact Fluorescent Lighting (CFL's) – You will recognize these lights by the bulbs that are spiral-shaped in appearance. They emit a lot of blue light, and they are a cause of concern for environmental groups related to their mercury content, and how to dispose of them safely. They became popular though as they are more energy efficient, and last longer than incandescent bulbs. These are the bulbs that take a while to get bright when switched on.

Light-Emitting Diodes (LED's) – These bulbs have become even more popular as they are even more energy efficient than CFL's, and they get bright immediately. However, regular LED light bulb scan emit blue light, and disrupt sleep patterns.

Fortunately, as science is proving the need to eliminate blue light before bedtime and during sleep, some companies are listening. General Electric, for example, has created their "GE Align" lighting. These particular LED's are designed so as not to disrupt the body's natural sleep rhythms. They do this by controlling how much blue light is emitted. They have AM bulbs meant to be like daylight, which helps to suppress melatonin production. On the other hand, the PM bulbs have an amber light that is similar to the light of candles and campfires. In this way, they do not disrupt your evening melatonin production needed for quality sleep.

Lighting Science is another company that takes pride in the creation of bulbs for both your home and your body. Its "Goodnight" Sleep-Enhancing bulbs use the same technology as was created for the NASA astronauts.

SCS Lighting Solutions, another company, create the "Sleep Ready Light Bulb," and offer the perfect option for your bedside lamp.

All of these bulbs are available for sale at places such as Amazon. In addition, most or all companies offer a daytime option, which can help increase your alertness when you wake up by suppressing melatonin production.

NINE

Better Sleep? Reduce the Temperature

"No day is so bad it can't be fixed with a nap." ~ Carrie Snow

Studies are showing that quality sleep is as important to your health as eating well, exercising, not smoking, and so forth. Sleep is a complex, restorative process. Your body controls the release of hormones and substances that help you sleep. However, many aspects of good sleep are also in your control and require your participation. The use of proper artificial lighting in your home is one way that you can control the quality of sleep you get every night. However, there are other things, related to your body's temperature that can also be done to prepare your body for a good night of sleep. In what follows, are some of those ideas?

Have you ever tried to sleep after a hot shower or bath, or even in a bedroom that is too warm? You undoubtedly know that this makes it more difficult to fall asleep, and it is also harder to remain sleeping.

In preparation for good sleep, your body's internal temperature must drop about a degree. This normally starts to occur around 90 to 120 minutes before sleep is to occur. Fortunately, in most circumstances, you can manipulate your body's temperature. Knowing this, here is what you need to do to allow this to happen:

- **Avoid hot showers and hot baths right before bed** – Keep the temperature of the water from warm to cool. In fact, in summer, take a cooler shower or go for a cool swim. If possible, go to bed with wet hair, as this will keep your body cooler and improve your sleep.

- **Avoid exercising right before bed** – This is something that you have always heard, but do you really know why this is an issue? It is because, not only does exercise stimulate you, it will also make you feel excessively warm to sleep. If possible, try to exercise earlier in the day. If that is not an option, and it often isn't for everyone, then you can help your body cool itself by taking a cool shower after your exercise workout.

- **Avoid excessive clothing before and at bedtime** – Another way to help your body cool down in the evenings, is to leave your arms and legs exposed. Think boxer shorts for guys, and light nightgowns for females. If you like wearing a fuzzy onesie to sleep, then reduce some of the bedding, or you will negatively affect your ability to fall asleep and to stay asleep.

- **Don't use hot water bottles and heating pads close to bedtime** – The same applies to too much bedding. In colder climates, if you want to warm up your bed before getting in, then put a heading pad in it for a few minutes before you get in, but then turn it off. Otherwise, its heat is bound to wake you up later.

- **Lower the temperature in your home** – With timers on thermostats, you can set the temperature in your home to be lowered a couple hours before bedtime. This will also help with reducing your core body temperature, making it easier to fall asleep, and stay asleep.

While you sleep, aim for a room temperature of no higher than 70 degrees F. 65 degrees F seems to be the most ideal, but you may have to experiment to find what suits your sleep the best.

TEN

Sleeping Pills? 3 Things to Consider First

"Laugh and the world laughs with you, snore and you sleep alone." ~ Anthony Burgess

Sleep is a natural process, but it seems so hard to get sometimes, and you may feel desperate. That is why the pharmaceutical companies keep coming up with new medications for sleep. However, sleeping medications (prescription and non-prescription) should not be your first go-to, if you suddenly find yourself having difficulty falling asleep or maintaining your sleep. This is a discussion that will need to occur with your medical doctor, who knows your medical history and lifestyle challenges.

Before deciding that sleeping pills are required, here are some things to ask yourself first:

1. Are you looking for short-term results?

Over-the-counter or prescription sleeping medications may help you in the short-term, but you are not really fixing the root cause of your sleeping problems. For example, sleeping medications may help with temporary issues such as jet lag, or adjusting to a shift change at work, but they should never be a long-term solution.

Of concern is that some sleeping medications result in dependence. The side effects of the medications can also be problematic. For example, the effects of the medication may not wear off before morning, making it unsafe to drive with the medication still in your body. Some people have also been known to do things while under the influence of sleeping medications, such as eating, texting, and even having sex while asleep!

2. Have you tried making lifestyle changes?

Many sleeping issues can be resolved or improved significantly simply by adjusting your lifestyle and your environment. For example, you can learn to control when and how much blue light exposure you get, thus affecting your sleep hormones. This applies to getting adequate daylight, and avoiding computer screens, tablets, etc. before bedtime.

You can also implement ways that bring your core body temperature down, a necessity to falling asleep. By using stress-reduction techniques, such as meditation, yoga, prayer and deep breathing exercises, you can also learn to sleep better. Other techniques include waking up at the same time every day, getting enough physical exercise in the day, and not drinking caffeine at least six hours before you go to sleep.

3. Have you tried natural supplements or essential oils for sleeping?

In addition to lifestyle and environmental changes mentioned above, natural supplements and essential oils that promote sleep exist. Because even natural products can exert strong biological effects, it is wise to consult with your physician before starting to use them, or better yet a pharmacist or a naturopathic doctor who can guide you on their use. This is especially important if you are using other herbal products or prescription medications. A nature-pathic doctor can be an invaluable resource to educating you on lifestyle habits, changes you can make, as well as the most appropriate suitable natural supplements and essential oils that may help you.

ELEVEN

Medical Conditions that Interfere with Sleep

"Tired minds don't plan well. Sleep first, plan later." – Walter Reisch

If you are always exhausted, despite making real attempts at improving your sleep, or you have trouble falling asleep or staying asleep (insomnia), then you should discuss this with your medical doctor and medical professional. There are two reasons for this. First, some medications contain compounds that make it harder to sleep. For example, some pain medications have caffeine in them. In addition, some asthma medications, and even nasal decongestants can also disrupt your sleep routine. This is just the tip of the iceberg. Second, a number of health conditions, both physical and mental, can interfere with your sleep, and some of them can actually be dangerous.

Here are a few physical medical conditions to know about.

Sleep Apnea – This is actually a very common sleep disorder. Unfortunately, sleep apnea is quite serious, as it involves the interruption of breathing during sleep. Pauses in breathing can last from a few seconds to much longer, and they can occur many times an hour. In one type of sleep apnea, the brain does not send the signals for breathing to occur.

The second type of sleep apnea is more common, and it is called "obstructive sleep apnea," because it involves the collapse of tissues in the throat during sleep. It is more common in overweight and obese individuals, and weight loss can be a solution to the problem. However, other things that can contribute to sleep apnea include large tonsils, sinus issues, family history, and so on. So even if you are not overweight, you can still be affected by sleep apnea. In fact, children are also diagnosed with sleep apnea.

Other risk factors for sleep apnea are:

- Being of male gender (most common)

- Being a smoker
- You have high blood pressure
- You have asthma
- You have diabetes
- You have reflux/heartburn
- You are older than 40
- You have nasal blockages from large adenoids, sinus problems, or the bone between your nostrils is offset (deviated nasal septum)

Some of the signs and symptoms that point to the possibility of sleep apnea include:

- Choking during sleep
- Loud snoring
- Morning headaches
- Pauses in your breathing while sleeping
- Dry mouth when waking up
- Exhausted
- High blood pressure
- Waking up with a dry throat

If you or your partner notice any of the above, be sure to speak to your medical professional.

In order to make a diagnosis, your doctor may order a **sleep lab test** or a **sleep home test** to confirm if sleep apnea is the source of your sleep woes. If sleep apnea is confirmed, then your doctor will determine the next step. People suffering from sleep apnea deal with not only the negative effects of sleep deprivation, but also the strain of trying to cope with oxygen deprivation at night. This puts serious strain on the brain, the heart, and the rest of the body.

As previously mentioned, weight loss may be recommended. If large tonsils or adenoids are the issue, then surgery may be the preferred treatment plan to clear air passages. Some people may benefit from special dental appliances or mouth guards that help keep their airway open during sleep. Smoking cessation can also help, as can ensuring you don't sleep on your back. Sometimes, a special machine such as a CPAP (Continuous Positive Airway Pressure) will be recommended to ensure that the tissues in your throat do not collapse during sleep.

Heartburn – Heartburn is the result of regurgitation of stomach contents, including stomach acid, back up your food pipe (the esophagus) that causes a burning pain in your chest. These acidic contents can reach the back of your throat, causing you to cough or choke and wake up during sleep.

Fortunately, some effective techniques exist to help you manage heartburn, and improve your sleep. These include:

- **Use a bed wedge** – You can find these in medical supply stores that sell all kinds of medical equipment. If they do not have one in stock, they can be ordered in. The purpose for the use of a bed wedge is to raise your upper body on an incline, making it harder for stomach contents to move against gravity. Regular pillows are not effective as you need to raise your chest too.

- **Sleep on your left side** – This is not always effective for people with severe reflux that results in heartburn, but it is worth a try as it works for many. Studies have shown that when you sleep on your left side, there is less chance of stomach contents travelling up your food pipe to your throat when compared to right side lying. Here are two easy sayings to help you remember what side to sleep on: "Right is wrong." or "Left is right."

- **Elevate the head of your bed** – The easiest way to do this is to elevate the head of your bed six inches higher than that of your feet. You can purchase items called "bed blocks" from any medical store, as these are often used by people with arthritis or hip replacements to raise their beds. In the case of heartburn and reflux, you only put the bed blocks under the head of the bed. Like the bed wedge, it makes it harder for stomach acid to make its way upwards against gravity.

- **Consult with your doctor and a pharmacist** – Just as some medications interfere with sleep, some medications also contribute to reflux, causing you to lose quality and quantity of sleep.

- **Lose a few pounds** – By losing weight, you can decrease the severity and frequency of reflux and heartburn.

- **Do not eat a large meal right before bedtime** – A small snack is okay to help improve sleep, however you should not be eating a large meal two to three hours before bedtime. Depending on what you eat before bed, it may take your body 2-3 hours to digest its late night snack. In addition, it's advisable to avoid foods that make your reflux worse. You may need to use a food diary to determine what they are, or you may already know what to avoid. Common culprits are carbonated beverages, coffee, tea, spicy foods, garlic, onions, and fatty fried foods. Meats are harder to digest late night and tend to take 2-3 hours to digest.

- **Quit smoking** – This is much easier said than done. As you know, the average smoker makes many attempts before achieving success. However, it's always worth seeing if giving up your smoking habit also improves your sleep and especially if accompanied by a reduction in reflux symptoms. Smoking is known to relax the muscles of your food pipe (esophagus), contributing to reflux.

Diabetes -

One reason why you may not be sleeping well, is that you have diabetes and do not even know it. According to the Centers for Disease Control and Prevention, 30 million Americans have diabetes, and 25% of them don't even know it!

Diabetes and poor sleep go hand in hand. People whose blood sugars are high due to diabetes, often spend a lot of time up at night having to urinate. They also may wake up with night sweats, or wake up due to feelings of low blood sugar (hypoglycemia). Constant thirst for water through-out the day is a common symptom of diabetes also.

Conversely, poor sleep also increases your risk of diabetes.

If you are diabetic, by eating properly during the day and evening, you can stabilize your blood sugars, so that you will be better able to sleep at night.

Arthritis – It is estimated that 80% of people with arthritis also suffer from sleep problems. Pain in joints can make it difficult to find a comfortable position to fall asleep and to remain sleeping. Please see my book **Arthritis Relief Now at Amazon** too, for natural and effective protocols to deal with all forms of arthritis.

Thyroid Problems –

Your thyroid is a butterfly-shaped gland found in your neck, and it secretes hormones. It has a major role in controlling your metabolism.

If your thyroid is not functioning properly, it is possible that you have developed an overactive thyroid (hyperthyroidism), or an underactive thyroid (hypothyroidism).

If your thyroid is overactive, it makes it difficult to fall asleep, and you may also experience night sweats.

If your thyroid is underactive, then you feel sleepy and cold all the time.

Your physician can do a blood test that determines how your thyroid is functioning by measuring your levels of thyroid hormones. Seek out a functional medicine doctor as well, before considering any surgical procedures. There are natural approaches today that weren't known just a few years ago.

Restless Legs Syndrome –

This disorder is really a neurological disorder that originates in the brain. However, it is considered a sleep disorder, as it interferes with sleep.

Symptoms include unpleasant, uncomfortable, or painful sensations in the legs that occur when inactive such as sitting or lying still. These sensations create an intense urge to move the legs, resulting in the name, "restless legs syndrome." Symptoms tend to be worse in the late afternoon and evenings, and most severe during the night when you are trying to sleep. As a result, you have difficulty falling asleep or staying asleep.

Interestingly, the symptoms can subside in the morning, which is when people affected by restless legs syndrome, can achieve their most restful sleep. In some, but not all cases, restless legs syndrome is related to another health condition, such as iron-deficiency anemia, diabetes, or peripheral neuropathy (numbness and pain that results from damage – usually due to diabetes - to nerves in your arms and legs).

Perimenopause, Menopause, and Post-Menopause –

Whether your body is just beginning to change (perimenopause), or has already gone through menopause, many women experienced disrupted sleep due to a change in hormone levels - less production of estrogen and progesterone. These sleep disruptions tend to affect the quality of sleep, not the time spent sleeping. Hot flashes, sweating, and drenched pajamas can wake women up from sleep, resulting in next-day sleepiness.

It usually starts in a woman's 40s, but can start in her 30s or even earlier. Perimenopause lasts up until menopause, the point when the ovaries stop releasing eggs. In the last one to two years of perimenopause, this drop in estrogen speeds up. At this stage, many women have menopause symptoms.

Insomnia is also a common complaint of women in this stage of their lives. Hormone replacement therapy is sometimes used, or you can opt for more natural supplements such as black cohosh.

Depression –

Difficulty sleeping can be a sign of depression. Lack of sleep can also make the depression worse, as it is more difficult to cope with daily stresses when you are tired.

In addition, some people with depression sleep much more, and yet still feel fatigued all the time.

The depression can occur on its own, or it can accompany other medical issues. For example, an underactive thyroid can exhibit depression as a symptom. People with arthritis may also experience depression related to the pain that negatively affects their daily functioning.

Anxiety –

Just as with depression, anxiety can cause difficulty sleeping, or lack of sleep can cause anxiety. People with ongoing insomnia are at increased risk of developing a diagnosed anxiety disorder.

TWELVE

Improve Your Sleep with These Natural Supplements

"Don't give up on your dreams so soon, sleep longer." Anon

Natural supplements can be an effective tool to improve your sleep, when used in combination with other components of sleep hygiene. As they can have a powerful effect on your body, always consult with a knowledgeable healthcare practitioner who can guide you as to their proper use, and can consider whether they may interfere with other health conditions you have or other medications you may be taking.

In what follows, are supplements that are commonly used to get a better night sleep. It is important to note, however, that the determination of which particular supplements will help your sleep, will depend on what is causing you to have sleep problems in the first place.

Medical and psychological causes for loss of sleep, should always be ruled out first by your physician.

Valerian root is a sedative herb that has used for centuries to address insomnia. You can find standardized extracts in health food stores and pharmacies. Take one to two capsules a half hour before bedtime.

Melatonin – This sleep hormone is made naturally by your brain, and it is released in response to darkness. It is what contributes to the feeling of sleepiness. However, exposure to artificial blue light in your home in the evenings from your light bulbs, computer, tablets, smartphones, and televisions, for example, is suppressing the release of this important sleep hormone. In this way, melatonin regulates your sleep/wake cycle. Keep in mind that as you get older, your body produces less melatonin.

Melatonin supplements are not recommended for everyone (ex. Pregnant or nursing moms), so be sure to check with your healthcare practitioner before use. Never give any sleep supplement to your child or teen without first consulting with his/her physician.

Melatonin can be useful for shift workers, people with jet lag, people who fall asleep too early or too late, and those who have trouble falling asleep or staying asleep. It is also beneficial for those who experience the winter blues (medically known as Seasonal Affective Disorder), and if you experience cluster headaches.

Melatonin supplements are sold over-the-counter in natural food health stores, as well as in pharmacies in North America. Like most supplements sold in North America, they are not regulated, so you may need to try various ones to find those that work best for you. To aid you in comparing and contrasting various melatonin supplements, it can be helpful to use a sleep diary. Record the time you feel sleepy, if you wake up at night, what time you wake up in the morning, how you feel (refreshed or not) when you wake up, and so forth.

You can also buy various doses of melatonin, as high as 10 mg, but do not assume that the more, the better. Higher doses are associated with morning grogginess, headaches, dizziness, vivid dreams and nightmares, and other side effects.

It is wiser to start with a lower dose, and adjust it upwards gradually, only if needed. This is where speaking and consulting with a healthcare professional, who is knowledgeable on the topic of sleep supplements, can help you tremendously.

In other words, there is no one solution for all. Studies are focusing on determining how much melatonin should be taken, and when to take it. Generally speaking though, between 2/10 of a mg and 5 mg supplementation 60 – 90 minutes before bedtime seems to work best for those using it. However, be prepared also to experiment with what time works best to take a certain dosage of melatonin. You do this by taking note of when that particular dose of melatonin starts to make you feel sleepy.

In addition to different doses of melatonin, pay attention to whether the brand you are trying is instant release. These are better if you have trouble falling asleep. However, if you have trouble staying asleep, you may find time-release melatonin more effective for you. Some people need a combination of both types, if they have trouble both falling and staying asleep.

As a hormone, melatonin regulates the wake/sleep cycle and other daily biorhythms. Try sublingual tablets (to be placed under the tongue and allowed to dissolve); take 2.5 mg at bedtime as an occasional dose, making sure that your bedroom is completely dark. A much lower dose, 0.25 to 0.3 mg, is more effective for regular use.

GABA and L-theanine – These are two supplements that will be spoken of together, because they have similarities in common, as well as differences.

L-theanine – This supplement is sold in health food stores, and over the counter in pharmacies. L-theanine is actually found naturally in tea leaves. It is an amino acid that has structural characteristics similar to glutamate, which is another amino acid in your body. Glutamate is a precursor to GABA. GABA is a chemical messenger in your brain that sends messages to other cells in your brain. GABA will be discussed in more detail a little bit later, but the important thing that you need to know now is that L-theanine increases the production of GABA.

A lot of research has been done with L-theanine, demonstrating that it can calm your mind, and increase concentration and focus, without causing drowsiness. It is also good for relaxation and reducing stress. Green tea contains the most L-theanine, but it is also found in black and oolong teas. It is not found in rooibos tea, which originates from a red bush native to South Africa. It is also not found in herbal teas, which are not made from tea leaves.

Research has also shown that L-theanine works harmoniously with caffeine. In other words, when you consume tea that contains both ingredients – L-theanine and caffeine – you will feel mentally more alert, calm, and less affected by the caffeine in the tea. This is unlike coffee, which only contains caffeine, and can make you feel jittery. Even if you decide to drink decaffeinated tea, you will still receive the benefits of the L-theanine as no difference exists in concentrations of L-theanine between caffeinated and decaffeinated versions. Choosing the decaffeinated version is the wiser option if you drink a lot of tea, or if you like to relax with a cup of tea in the evening before going to bed.

L-theanine is relatively safe, but it can lower blood pressure, so as with anything, always speak to your doctor and pharmacist before using.

GABA – This is short for gamma-amino-butyric acid, but for simplicity sake, it's called GABA. Like already mentioned, GABA is a chemical made by your brain that sends messages to other cells (it's a neurotransmitter) in your brain. Like L-theanine, it provides a calming and relaxing effect on your cells. Unlike L-theanine, however, it is not found in tea. As mentioned previously though, GABA's precursor, glutamate or glutamic acid, is found in food.

Examples of foods that contain the precursor to GABA include ripe tomatoes, walnuts, kefir, sea vegetables, tree nuts, bananas, citrus fruits (oranges), brown rice, and fermented vegetables such as sauerkraut. By including more GABA-producing foods in your diet, you can actually increase the amount of GABA in your brain, which will allow you to relax and feel calmer.

Vitamin B6 is also very important in the production of GABA.

Related to this, studies have shown that less GABA is found in the brains of people who suffer from insomnia. Therefore, sufficient levels of GABA in your brain appear important in ensuring that you fall asleep easily, as well as have a refreshing sleep. Without enough GABA, deep, restorative sleep is not possible.

GABA supplements do not appear to be absorbed readily by the body, and it is possible to overdose on GABA supplements. Therefore, if you want to increase your GABA levels, foods that help produce it (like those mentioned above), are probably your best bet.

L-theanine works in collaboration with GABA by improving GABA's effectiveness in calming your mind.

B Vitamins – The B vitamins play an important role in many functions within your body. The eight B vitamins – B1 (Thiamine), B2 (Riboflavin), B3 (Niacin), B5 (Pantothenic Acid), B6 (Pyridoxine), B7 (Biotin), B9 (Folate), and B12 (Cobalamins) – are known as the B-complex.

Although each of the B vitamins has its own role, they still work together. Vitamins B3, B5, B6, B9, and B12, in particular, play an important role in sleep quality. For example, if you are deficient in Vitamin B6, your body produces less GABA, which is an important chemical messenger known for relaxation and calmness in the brain for sleep.

Vitamin B12 is another "sleep vitamin" that helps in the production of melatonin (the sleep hormone) required for good sleep. Vitamin B9 is also important for those people who suffer from a condition known as "restless legs syndrome" during sleep.

Magnesium – This mineral plays an important role in your mood, metabolism, maintenance of your bone and heart health, as well as promotion of healthy sleep. Magnesium is also involved in your body's reaction to stress, and it is helpful in reducing anxiety as well. Insomnia has also been linked to low magnesium levels. Magnesium plays an important role in ensuring you enter the deep, restorative stage of sleep. In addition, magnesium increases levels of GABA – the chemical in your brain that produces a calming effect on your cells so that you can fall asleep. This is just a small sampling and explanation of how important it is to have adequate levels of magnesium in your body at all times.

Magnesium is not produced by your body. Therefore, you must get it in food sources or through supplements. Food sources include dark leafy vegetables, dairy, broccoli, almonds, sunflower seeds, and others. Unfortunately, many people do not get enough magnesium through their diets alone. It is estimated that **eighty** percent of Americans are not getting enough magnesium and may be deficient. As a result, supplementation may be required. Always speak to a physician knowledgeable in sleep disorders, a naturopathic doctor, and/or pharmacist to provide you with advice as to whether you should be supplementing with magnesium.

This is especially important if you have any pre-existing health conditions, or if you are already on medications as magnesium can potentially interact with them. The healthcare practitioner will also be able to provide you with a dosage level, if it is determined that you would benefit from magnesium. Magnesium citrate is absorbed decently, and is a better option over magnesium oxide which is not.

Dr. Michael J. Breus, PhD. The Sleep Doctor™ thesleepdoctor.com has an amazing article on the benefits of 5-HTP, a supplement that can really help.

Many people have tried 5-HTP for emotional issues, and others have tried it for sleep. Here, I do a review of 5-HTP so we can all learn a little more about this fascinating supplement.

Most of us have experienced how emotional distress can lead to restless, sleepless nights and difficult days. Whether it's a tough break up, a tricky situation at work, or a more prolonged struggle with depression or anxiety, our emotions and stress levels can throw sleep off kilter.

There's complicated relationship between mood and sleep—depression, anxiety and stress can interfere with healthy sleep, and poor sleep makes us more vulnerable to problems with mood and emotional regulation.

The compound 5-HTP has effects on both sleep and mood, as well as other body functions that impact our health and our ability to feel good during the day and sleep restfully at night. Let's take a closer look at what this mood-boosting, sleep-promoting compound does in the body, the benefits it may have for sleep, health, and quality of life.

What is 5-HTP?

5-Hydroxytryptophan—commonly known as 5-HTP—is a compound made naturally in the body. 5-HTP is created as a by-product of the amino acid L-tryptophan. Our bodies don't make L-tryptophan naturally—we absorb this essential amino acid from the foods we eat.

5-HTP is produced as a supplement from the seeds of a plant, Griffonia simplicfolia, which is native to West Africa. As we age, natural levels of 5-HTP appear to decline.

How does 5-HTP work?

5-HTP helps the body to produce more serotonin. Serotonin is a neurotransmitter that plays a key role in regulating mood and sleep-wake cycles. Healthy levels of serotonin contribute to a positive mood and outlook and also promote restful sleep. Serotonin also plays an important role in many other of the body's functions, including digestion, appetite, and pain perception.

Serotonin influences sleep and sleep-wake cycles in many ways, and scientists continue to make discoveries about how this important neurochemical affects our sleeping and waking lives. One important way serotonin affects sleep and bio time is through its relationship with the "sleep hormone" melatonin. Melatonin is made from serotonin in the presence of darkness. (Remember, melatonin production in the body is triggered by darkness and suppressed by exposure to natural and artificial light.) Healthy serotonin levels are essential for maintaining healthy melatonin levels—and both serotonin and melatonin are critical to sleep and a well-functioning bio clock. With its ability to increase serotonin, 5-HTP supports a neurochemical process that can enable high-quality sleep and keep the body's bio clock in sync.

Because of its serotonin-boosting capability, 5-HTP may also help with other conditions, including mood problems, stress, pain, and appetite control.

Benefits of 5-HTP

Sleep and sleep-wake cycles

Because of its role in creating serotonin, 5-HTP is indirectly involved in producing melatonin, a hormone that is critical for sleep. Melatonin helps the body's bio clock stay in sync, and regulates daily sleep-wake cycles. A strong bio clock and regular sleep-wake routines are the cornerstone of healthy, restful, rejuvenating sleep. Research suggests that 5-HTP may help shorten the time it takes to fall asleep and increase sleep amounts.

5-HTP can be effective in improving mood, and easing symptoms of stress and anxiousness, which can in turn interfere with sleep.

Research also indicates that 5-HTP may be effective in helping to reduce sleep terrors in children.

Stress, anxiety, and depression 5-HTP has been shown in scientific studies to promote relaxation and alleviate stress and anxiety. The relaxation and anti-anxiety properties of 5-HTP appear to come from its ability to elevate levels of serotonin. Research has demonstrated that 5-HTP may reduce the risks of panic attacks and symptoms of panic, as well as anxiety and emotional stress. Research also indicates 5-HTP may be effective in helping to alleviate depression.

Appetite suppression and weight control for decades, 5-HTP has been recognized as important to appetite regulation. Higher levels of serotonin are linked to diminished appetite. Keeping serotonin levels from dipping can help keep appetite in check, and may help reduce cravings for carbohydrates. As a serotonin booster, 5-HTP may help to suppress appetite. Research indicates that 5-HTP may be effective in helping people who are overweight or obese lose weight.

Fibromyalgia

Fibromyalgia is a condition that often combines chronic physical pain with sleep problems. Research indicates that 5-HTP can help improve fibromyalgia symptoms, including pain, tenderness, daytime fatigue, sleep quality, and anxiety.

Migraines and headache pain

There's scientific evidence indicating that 5-HTP may be able to reduce the frequency of migraine headache attacks and reduce pain from chronic headaches.

Other uses for 5-HTP

Because of its direct influence over serotonin and indirect influence over other hormones including melatonin, scientists are investigating the therapeutic potential for 5-HTP for a range of conditions, including:

- Menopausal symptoms
- Premenstrual dysphoric disorder (PMDD)
- Premenstrual syndrome (PMS)
- Attention deficit-hyperactivity disorder (ADHD)
- Parkinson's disease
- Alzheimer's disease
- Nervous system disorder
- Ramsey-Hunt syndrome
- Alcohol and drug withdrawal symptoms

5-HTP: what to know

Always consult your doctor before you begin taking a supplement or make any changes to your existing medication and supplement routine. This is not medical advice, but it is information you can use as a conversation-starter with your physician at your next appointment.

5-HTP dosing

The following doses are based on amounts that have been investigated in scientific studies. In general, it is recommended that users begin with the smallest suggested dose, and gradually increase until it has an effect.

A range of doses from 25mg to 500mg and higher has been studied in scientific research, for sleep problems, anxiety, depression, stress, appetite suppression, and other conditions.

Possible side effects of 5-HTP

5-HTP is generally well tolerated by healthy adults. Possible side effects of 5-HTP include stomach pain, nausea, vomiting, diarrhea, heartburn, excessive sleepiness, muscle spasms, and sexual problems.

People with the following conditions should consult with a physician before using a 5-HTP supplement:

• **Pregnancy** and breast feeding
• **Surgery patients** (Some surgery medications can affect serotonin. It's generally recommended that people stop taking 5-HTP at least two weeks ahead of

scheduled surgery.)

• **Children.** Talk with your child's physician before beginning your child's use of 5-HTP.

5-HTP has been linked in very rare instances to a condition known as EMS, or eosinophilia-myalgia syndrome, which combines extreme muscle tenderness with abnormalities in the blood. A contaminant that was found in some tryptophan supplements in the late 1980s, and was linked to a small number of EMS cases, was also found in some 5-HTP supplements. It's important to talk with your doctor before you begin taking 5-HTP or any other supplement, and to make sure you're getting your supplements from a reliable provider.

5-HTP interactions

The following medications and other supplements may interact with 5-HTP. Effects may include increasing or decreasing sleepiness and drowsiness, interfering with the effectiveness of the medications or supplements, and interfering with the condition that is being treated by the medication or supplement. These are lists of commonly used medications and supplements that have scientifically identified interactions with 5-HTP. People who take these or any other medications and supplements should consult with a physician before beginning to use 5-HTP.

Interactions with medications:

• Carbidopa (used to treat Parkinson's disease)
• Dextromethorphan (found in cough medicines including Robitussin DM and others)
• Antidepressant medications
• MAOIs
• Pain medications (including Demerol, Talwin, Tramadol and others)
• Sedative medications

Interactions with other supplements:

Using 5-HTP in combination with other herbs or supplements that may cause sleepiness or drowsiness may lead to excessive sleepiness. These herbs and supplements include but are not limited to:

- Calamus
- California poppy
- Catnip
- Hops
- Jamaican dogwood
- Kava
- St. John's Wort
- Skullcap
- Valerian
- Yerba mansa

Using 5-HTP in combination with other herbs or supplements that increase serotonin levels may lead to too-high of serotonin levels. These herbs and supplements include but are not limited to:

- Hawaiian baby wood rose
- L-tryptophan
- S-adenosylmethionine (SAMe)
- St. John's Wort

Emotional balance and management of stress levels and mood make an enormous difference to sleep, as well as to performance, quality of life, and overall health. If these issues interfere with your sleep and your daily well-being, consider speaking with your doctor about whether 5-HTP might help.

Essential Oils have a real place in treating insomnia as well. Practioners have been recommending oils for years. Here are a few that sufferers have had great success with. From Prairie Homestead here are a few.

8 Essential Oils for Sleep

- Lavender. I'm betting you probably aren't surprised to see lavender at the top of the list, huh?
- Vetiver. It essential oil is distilled from the roots of the plant.
- Roman Chamomile
- Ylang Ylang
- Bergamot
- Sandalwood
- Marjoram
- Cedarwood

There are two methods that are used with oils

1. Topical Use

Applying oil topically can be a wonderful way to reap their benefits. You generally rub oils on the back of my neck, or on the bottoms of my feet before bed. You can usually use a vegetable oil of some sort (*like sweet almond oil*– *affiliate link*) to dilute them, and then rub them into your skin.

2. Aromatic Use

Another secret essential oil weapon is essential oil diffusers. If you are having a hard time deciding on a diffuser, It's easy to add just a few drops of any of these oils to a bit of water in your essential oil diffuser, set by your bedside, and you'll be in dreamland in no time.

There are new essential oil companies popping up every day, but I've used and recommended doTERRA essential oils for years now, and love them,. The oils are third-party tested for purity and ethically sourced around the globe. doTERRA oils just work better. Give them a shot.

INTERMISSION

The Top 30 Most Famous Insomniacs

"I've got a bad case of the 3:00 am guilt's - you know, when you lie in bed awake and replay all those things you didn't do right? Because, as we all know, nothing solves insomnia like a nice warm glass of regret, depression and self-loathing."
— *D.D. Barant, Dying Bites*

Let's take a little break shall we? If you lie awake at night tossing and turning, take heart. Somewhere out there, you have great company. From Celebrities. Politicians. Artists, Singers and your next door neighbor.

Below is a list of the top 30 greatest insomniacs of all time--some still alive and some resting in peace at last--along with either their personal tips on how to sleep or the problems lack of sleep caused in their lives.

The top 30 most famous insomniacs of all time:

1. Arianna Huffington, founder of The Huffington Post. She once got so little sleep that she passed out from exhaustion, breaking her cheekbone. Since then, Huffington is a fervent anti-insomnia crusader, declaring lack of sleep a feminist issue. She has even installed napping rooms for employees in her workplace. Still living.

2. Vincent Van Gogh, painter. Don't try this at home, kids, but Van Gogh treated his insomnia by dousing his mattress and pillow with camphor, which is related to turpentine. Historians think this may have slowly poisoned him and factored into his suicide. He died at

3. Bill Clinton, president. The former president of the United States, who famously slept just five hours a night, partly blames his heart attack on fatigue.

4. Marilyn Monroe, actress, model, singer. Her insomnia, which may have been linked to her emotional turbulence, was treated with sleeping pills. The day before she overdosed and died, she was reportedly enraged when she heard a friend had slept for 15 hours. Monroe died at 36.

5. Bill Clinton, president. Bill Clinton used to proudly speak of only needing five hours of sleep per night, but since his heart operations, he has changed his routine.

6. Madonna, singer. Madonna's brother, Christopher Ciccone, dished on his famous sister, insisting that she blames her insomnia on an "unbridled desire for fame and fortune." Madonna treats it with medication.

7. Judy Garland, actress. When she was only a teenager, the movie studio demanded she stay thin. Garland became addicted to amphetamines, which she says caused her insomnia--keeping her awake for three or four days at a time. Judy died at 47.

8. Groucho Marx, comic actor. Marx says it was the 1929 stock market crash that triggered his insomnia. When he couldn't sleep, he would do one of two things: call strangers on the phone and insult them or he would write jokes. One such joke, written in the middle of the night.
Q: What do you get when you cross an insomniac, an

agnostic and a dyslexic? **A:** Someone who stays up all night wondering if there is a Dog. Groucho died at 86.

9. Margaret Thatcher, politician. As the British prime minister, Thatcher slept just four hours a night, saying, "Sleep is for wimps." Thatcher died at 87.

10. Tallulah Bankhead, actress. This early 20th century film star and libertine solved her insomnia by hiring gay "caddies" to sit with her and hold her hand until she fell asleep. She died at 66.

11. George Clooney, actor. Clooney suffers from insomnia and he claims that leaving the television on helps him fall asleep.

12. Sandra Bullock, actress. Sandra Bullock suffers from insomnia. 'I have been surprised by the fact that I really only need 3 hours of sleep,' she says. She often hides her tired eyes behind sunglasses.

13. Michael Jackson, musician. Famous insomniacs have actually died as a result of their condition. Michael Jackson overdosed on the medication propofol, which he was using it as a sleep aid. Michael died at 50 years old.

14. **Vincent van Gogh, painter**. Van Gogh was a true insomniac. He used to pour a turpentine-like liquid on his mattress to help him sleep. He died at 37.

15. **Anna Nicole Smith, model, actress**. Anna was an insomniac, and an overdose of sleeping medication contributed to her death. She died at 40.

16. **Napoleon Bonaparte. French leader.** Historians state that Napoleon Bonaparte was an insomniac especially during times of great stress. Napoleon died at 51.

17. **Heath Ledger, actor.** Heath Ledger suffered from exhaustion and insomnia, and sleeping pills were a factor in his early death. He died at 29.

18. **Simon Cowell, reality television judge and producer.** Simon used hypnosis to treat his insomnia.

19. **Lady Gaga, musician**. Lady Gaga says that she has trouble sleeping because her music is always on her mind.

20. **Abraham Lincoln, president.** Abraham Lincoln used to treat his insomnia by taking long walks

in the middle of the night. Lincoln was shot and died at 56.

21. Cary Grant, actor. Cary Grant suffered from insomnia and he would frequently get up in the middle of the night and read. He died at 82.

22. Benjamin Franklin, statesman, inventor, founding father. Franklin suffered from insomnia and he even had two beds he alternated between to try and help his condition. Franklin died at 84.

23. Theodore Roosevelt, president. Roosevelt used to drink cognac before bed to treat his insomnia. Died at 61.

24. Jimi Hendrix, musician. Hendrix was rumored to have insomnia and died from an overdose of sleep medication. Died at 27.

25. Margaret Thatcher, Prime Minister of Great Britain. Thatcher was a well-known insomniac. She had the motto, "sleep is for wimps." Died at 88.

26. Mark Twain Author. Mark Twain suffered from insomnia and died at 74. He famously said, "Don't go to sleep, so many people die there." And "the secret to getting ahead is getting started."

27. Jessica Simpson, singer. Jessica Simpson claims that sleeping on the floor helps her fall asleep when she is suffering from insomnia.

28. W.C. Fields, actor. W.C. Fields was an insomniac, and he could only sleep if he heard the sounds of rain. He eventually got a large umbrella and attached a sprinkler to it to emulate the sound of rain. He dies at 66.

29. Charles Dickens, writer. Author Charles Dickens would walk the streets of London when he was suffering from insomnia. He died at 58.

30. Marlene Dietrich, actress. Actress Marlene Dietrich used natural sleep remedies to treat her insomnia. She dies at 91.

11 ENERGIZING TRICKS & HACKS

To Get You Back On Track

"In the morning I can't eat, I'm thinking of you. In the evening I can't eat, I'm thinking of you. In the night I can't sleep, I'm so hungry!" ~Anon

Limit your options for less indecision

Most people feel as if they don't have enough time in the day. They end up working into the late evening hours either at work or at their "second shift" at home. Often, this means they are missing out on a lot of time that should be used resting, sleeping, and re-energizing.

Schedule Everything

The way that you can prevent this problem is through scheduling and limiting your options. Use an online calendar or a paper calendar - either is fine. Take a blank one-week calendar with 168 hours on it. Now fill-in every appointment that shows up weekly in your week and fill that in first. This includes your weekly work schedule, 7-8 hours of sleep, doctor's appointments, church times, your early morning wake-up routine, date night with your spouse on Friday nights, family time, sporting events and practices, etc.

Now you have a real idea of how much time you really have left to do other things. Probably not much, right? When I did this exercise myself, I realized that I only had 34 hours a week to myself, to really do the things I wanted to do. It's pretty eye-opening. But, when you really know how busy you are, it can help you make better decisions. Now when someone else asks you to put something else on your plate, you can look at your calendar and decide if it's possible. Then it's easier to say no because there's just no room on your calendar.

Cut Down on Choices

The next thing to do is to cut down on other types of choices. For example, if you plan your meals in advance, you won't have to stand there for 20 minutes trying to figure out what's for dinner. Instead, you simply look at your weekly meal plan on the fridge each morning, take out what needs to be thawed, prepare anything in advance that you can, and dinner will be on the table faster and with less hassle and stress.

Another thing that can take a lot of time is figuring out what to wear. If you lay out your clothing the night before, throw out things you never wear, and only have one black dress pant and one black boot, it will take a lot less time - not only getting ready but also cleaning your clothes. Most of us have far too many things, and duplicates at that, which causes us to take too much time choosing, cleaning, and organizing. Simplifying save times money and frustration. Set a date every 3-6 months where you create a "Simplify Our Life" Saturday, where you regularly go through your house and do a purge of things that no longer serve you. It's regenerating. It reduces stress, and the promise is that you'll sleep so much better with this tweak in your calendar.

When you know what you have, and everything has a place, it's easier to tell what you need more of and what you need less of. You'll save not only money but time and frustration. And when you save time that gives you something very precious that you cannot get more of and is truly priceless. When you save money, you save having to be stressed out because of lack of money. It's a win-win all the way around.

So remember the goal...is to help you to get more sleep at night and give you more energy every day with less stress.

Power off your electronics and give yourself a break

Due to the advent of electronics like mobile devices, tablets, and computers (not to mention streaming TV), insomnia seems to have risen to epidemic proportions. People honestly do believe they're getting more done because they think they're multitasking. They're watching TV, talking to people on social media, checking their work email, and shopping all at once, instead of relaxing as they should be.

This isn't helping you at all. The truth is, all you're doing is destroying your circadian rhythm. Humans need light and dark at certain times in order to feel well rested and energetic throughout the day.

The Circadian Rhythm

A circadian rhythm is an internal 24-hour clock that all humans have. It's always running and is always aware. It can get out of whack due to artificial lighting in your home, in addition to the electronics we use such as mobile devices, televisions, and computer screens. Essentially, all screens can interfere with your cycle if you aren't careful. Some people are more susceptible to problems than others. But everyone is affected one way or another - even if it's just having your mind being stimulated 24/7 without a break.

It's important to remember, in terms of energy, that peaks and valleys throughout the day are normal. Almost everyone experiences the 3 pm slump and almost everyone experiences that time before the slump that happens several hours after waking for the day, when they are at peak performance getting work done very fast. Ideally, you want to learn and understand your circadian rhythm and how it works so you can be most energetic during the time you need to be.

The Benefit of Turning off Your Electronics

One way to avoid affecting your natural 24-hour rhythm is to start turning off electronics at least an hour or two before bedtime. If you want to go to bed at 10 pm, then you'll want to shut your electronics and television down by 8 to 9 pm each evening. This can be difficult for some people because those are prime TV watching hours. But, it's okay because today you can record everything or watch it at a different time using streaming services. Your sleep cycle is more important, and you can watch those shows any time you want to. Make your bedtime a priority. A few minutes before or after your bedtime is okay, but keeping your commitment to yourself where sleep is concerned is crucial for relaxation, rejuvenation and long-term health.

Not only will shutting down pay off in terms of your family relationships, it will also help you find time to take care of yourself and get more sleep. After a good night's rest, that you planned for and executed, you're going to feel a lot more rested, more energized and will be more productive as well.

If you want to improve your life in a big way, this is one thing that will make a huge difference. Besides, wouldn't it be nice to be able to give each thing you do 100 percent attention rather than always having to check your phone or computer for another social media post or email? Try it for at least 14 days to see how invigorated you'll feel.

Cool your body to invigorate your mind

It's amazing what a difference temperature can make when you're trying to be mentally productive. It may seem strange to cool down to get more mental clarity and energize your mind, but it's all scientific. Think about this. Your brain uses glucose to run and cooling down tends to release the glucose, thus waking up your brain. Plus, you tend to burn more fat if you stay cooler than if you're hot and sluggish.

If you're feeling sluggish, try any of these cool-down methods to invigorate your mind and get back on track.

* **Yawning** – One reason your body is often triggered to yawn is due to the need for an extra kick of oxygen. But at the same time it cools your body down, thus enabling you to think more clearly. You can make yourself yawn by looking at a video of someone yawning, or by simply opening your mouth as if you're going to yawn until it happens.

* **Yoga** – There is a form of breathing in yoga called Sitali breath. This is simply breathing in through your mouth using your tongue as a type of filter. Just stick your tongue out and curl it into "U" shape. Then sitting comfortably with good posture breathe in through your mouth and out through your nose with a long inhale and a slow exhale. Do this about ten times to cool down. Great desk activity to do when you're experiencing the 3 pm slump.

* **Turn Down the Thermostat** – If possible, make your room cooler at night for sleeping. The ideal sleeping temperature is between 60 and 68 degrees

Fahrenheit. If you can manage to cool your room down like that, you'll sleep much better and wake up more invigorated.

* **Eat Fruit** – An ideal daytime snack about 30 minutes before your normal slump time is to eat some form of berry. Strawberries, raspberries, and cherries are all good choices to eat. Alternatively, you can eat any type of fruit you want that is low in fat and high in moisture to cool down, including melons, even bananas. If you want to avoid too much sugar, however, try cucumbers.

* **Stay Hydrated** – One of your best weapons against brain fog is water. Notice I didn't say a coffee or a soda pop. These drinks slam you down an hour later and mess with your natural sleep rhythms. Try to keep water with you throughout your day. The best temperature for water is really room temperature or just slightly cooler. You don't need to make it super-cold because then your body has to work harder to get it to the right temperature, which could make you hotter. How much water? Shoot for half your body weight in ounces. For example, a 150-pound woman

should drink 75 ounces throughout the day. Don't guzzle the water; you want to work toward a slow drip to stay cool. Consider a higher pH alkaline water for complete body saturation as well. An 8.8 or 9.5 pH water quickly satisfies that constant thirstiness on hot days too.

* **Use Face Mist** – You can use filtered or alkaline water, but you can also buy face mist with essential oils that are energizing and safe. When you feel as if you cannot focus or concentrate, simply mist your face with the mineral water solution. Take the time to also breathe in deeply between sprays to give your body a little extra oxygen kick, which will also cool you down. The mineral water mist also gives your skin and hair a nutrient boost.

* **Change Your Socks** – This may sound a little strange but anytime you get hot and sweaty, even if you cool off later, your feet will often stay hot if you have the same socks on. The best way to give yourself a fast pick-up is to bring extra socks anytime you know you're going to work out physically to a sweat, then change them so that you can cool off faster.

If you want to increase your productivity or anyone's productivity, turn down the AC (or open the window if it's cool outside) to get the temperature down. A perfect daytime non-sleeping temperature is no hotter than 72 degrees F. Someplace between 68 and 72 degrees is best for keeping your brain energized.

Stretch Your Muscles

Have you ever watched a dog or a cat get up from their spot and stretch? They do it every single time they change positions. Believe it or not, if you copy your pet and start stretching gently any time you change positions, feel tired, or need energy, you'll invigorate your brain and feel better throughout the day. Muscles need to be stretched. Every waking hour, get up and move 5-10 minutes. You'll see as an inconvenience at first, and then recognize its value later as it shows up in your health.

The Benefits of Stretching

Aside from getting more energy, stretching provides many benefits, such as more flexibility, better posture, helps prevent injury, and helps get blood to your muscles which helps reduce soreness. In terms of your mind, obviously less pain is going to be uplifting, but stretching also calms you down, releases tension, and increases good energy so that you can be more productive. If you're at work, take a restroom break and spend a minute doing 50 side-to-sides for stretching. Literally slide your hands down your right then left side. It will energize you and keep you flexible too.

Stretch like Your Pet

If you want to add stretching to your day, think like a dog or a cat and do it every time you change positions or get tired. Especially stretch before and after exercises. Be careful stretching too much when your muscles aren't warm, though, and likewise be careful stretching too far just because you are warmed up. Stretching should never cause pain; it should feel good. Therefore, don't bounce a stretch and only move as far as feels natural to you.

If you want to learn more about stretching, consider signing up for yoga or a Pilate's class too. There you can learn about proper form so that you don't injure yourself. Some gyms now offer stretching (and yoga) classes, which is also a good way to learn proper techniques. You can also learn online via streaming classes through Lastics.com (https://lastics.com/). They use stretching techniques that dancers use to be flexible, elongate their muscles, and experience less pain.

Stretching in Your Chair

You can also stretch in your chair at the office. Occasionally, anytime you feel tired or strained, simply stand up, stand with your feet shoulders' width apart, put your hands on the small of your back, lean back slowly to arch your back just until you feel a very slight stretch in your abdominal muscles. It should not hurt. Hold for up to 20 seconds and repeat three times.

You can try many different chair exercises that mostly involve stretching, to help get the flow of blood to your brain and to your muscles. This will provide a tremendous boost of energy. If you need ideas, you can order a DVD from Amazon or look on Amazon for streaming choices. For example, Sit and Be Fit: Easy Fitness for Seniors by Mary Ann Wilson is a great choice, whether you're a senior or not. It will help you get through a sedentary day in the office.

Boost your circadian rhythms with sunlight

Sunlight is one of our most important natural resources for boosting your energy. But, sadly, due to how our schools, stores, and office buildings are made, many of us hardly ever see the sunlight. That can interfere with your natural circadian rhythms. If you're having trouble sleeping at night, getting really tired during the day, can't get up in the morning, or are lacking energy, you may want to consider sunlight therapy.

It's super-simple; get at least 45 minutes of sunlight each morning before 10 am. But there are many other factors that can help. Let's look at a few.

* Stick to a Schedule

Get up and go to bed at the same time each day, shooting for eight hours of sleep each night. Even if you go to a party Friday night, try to get up at the same time on Saturday morning or try not to make that a regular part of your week. Sticking as close to possible to the same schedule is going to help you feel more energetic every day, and will boost your circadian rhythms.

* Walk in the Morning

I've been doing this for years and it's really paid off. So I encourage you to get your steps in, and the best time to do that is in the morning. A quick, brisk 20-30-minute walk each morning when the sun comes up is going to do more for your ability to be energetic throughout the day than almost anything else you can do. Make it a game and do it regularly.

* Turn off Technology in the Evening

As least one to two hours before you plan to go to bed to sleep, turn off your electronics. The light from the screens can mess up your circadian rhythm and prevent your brain from wanting to go to sleep for several hours after you lie down. If you get a jump on it and turn down the lights, you'll go to sleep at a more regular time.

If you notice that it's hard for you to get in that walk, you can also get a "happy light." Set it on your desk for up to 45 minutes at least three or four times a week before 9 or 10 am, to trigger your mind to think it's sunlight.

Want to know why your mom was right that your posture matters?

Proper Posture Makes You Feel Energized

Did you know that something as simple as your posture can make you feel more energized? If you ever feel down, depressed, or just tired, think about what your posture is like. More than likely your posture is not that great. You're probably sitting with your shoulders slumped, resting your face on your hands, and generally lacking energy with every part of your body.

If you want to feel better immediately, try to train yourself to have good posture. Sitting up or standing up tall helps you breathe better, gets more oxygen into your lungs, and improves your mood in amazing ways. It's a lot like smiling. When you smile as you talk, it's hard to be mad or depressed even if you started out that way too.

Tips on Getting Your Posture Right

With your posture, if you're standing tall, you can be sure that you'll feel more energetic and more confident. It's amazing, but when you do this you slow down the release of cortisol into your blood and increase the number of red blood cells that get to the various parts of your body - including your brain. This will automatically give you more energy.

Try to set up a way to remind yourself to check your posture. One way to do this is to set up an alarm on your computer if you're at your desk all day as a reminder. Another way is to pick something that you often look at in the room to help remind you to check your posture.

Try putting down the mobile devices while you're doing other things so that you look up instead of down.

(This is a really common condition today called text neck). For example, when you go outside for a walk, don't look at your phone the entire time. Walk, look around, and keep your head up high. Even if you're exercising on your stationary bike, instead of looking at a book or your mobile device, look up, keeping your ribs open and your spine aligned, and you'll notice you are much more energetic.

When you're watching TV you can keep your posture positive by not multitasking and setting your television up in the right spot so that you can look at it comfortably straight ahead. Every little thing you can adjust to avoid slouching, avoid looking down, and avoid bending your neck down will help you get more energy into your day. Another key idea to regain your proper posture is to stretch your neck in the opposite direction through a neck orthotic or a folded towel that you place under the crook of your neck for 10-20 minutes a day, 3-4 times a week. The idea is to reshape your neck (like braces do for your teeth) can reduce stress and your forward head posture. Try it. It actually works very effectively.

Deep Breathing Gets Your Blood Pumping

It may seem strange, but most of us don't breathe correctly. Most of us are walking around breathing very shallowly, which can also make us very tired. It's also why starting around age four you lose your ability to be very loud. The main ingredient to more energy besides water is oxygen. To get more oxygen, you'll want to learn more about deep breathing and why it's so important for keeping you energized.

Watch an infant breathing. They breathe in and their tummy expands, they breathe out and their tummy contracts. An older person tends to move their chest in and out instead. So now that you know that, understand that you can practice deep diaphragmatic breathing to get your blood pumping and feel more energetic.

Follow These Directions:

Sit up straight in a hard-back chair and place a hand on your stomach. Now inhale through your nose deeply, filling your stomach region with air instead of your chest area. It might take a few tries to get it right. Keeping your hand on your stomach can help you focus. Your chest should not rise, but your stomach and lower ribs should expand. Then breathe out through your mouth, letting the air collapse your stomach and lower ribs. Do this slowly, deeply, about five to ten times.

Try to do this throughout the day so that you can train your body to mostly breathe diaphragmatically. This type of breathing will provide more oxygen to your organs - especially your digestive organs, which will improve digestion. When you have better digestion, you'll feel a lot more energetic.

Another way to accomplish this is to exercise aerobically. One of the best ways to do this is by jumping up and down on a mini-trampoline, also known as a rebounder. Rebounding helps you avoid damage to your joints but also enables you to work out aerobically, which is a great way to get your blood pumping to get all the vital nutrients to your important organs so that you can feel more energized throughout the day.

Aside from oxygen, the other thing you need is water. Over 75 percent of Americans suffer from dehydration. Learn the signs, effects, and how to avoid it next time. The accepted rule of thumb is, that if your lips are dried out, you're likely a third dehydrated already. Keep water handy at all times.

Employ Healing Frequencies

There have been a few studies of the effectiveness of frequencies on the mind and body. May I suggest, though it's an electronic device which we'd like to normally eliminate at bedtime that you experiment with 432 Hz frequency music for sleeping and deep relaxation several hours before bed.

Frequency is the term used to explain the rate at which all things vibrate. All matter is energy. Everything has a vibration frequency, which can be measured in Hertz (Hz). These electromagnetic frequencies have been researched for over a hundred years. In diagnostic medicine, frequencies are well known; EKG's for the heart, EEG's for the brain, and MRI's for injured cells. Complimentary medicine also uses frequencies, which are commonly being incorporated in cold laser therapy equipment as a suitable means of delivery to the cells and tissues of people, pets and plants, and also frequency associated with music and vibration are finding success in users to fight insomnia and overcome chronic sleep problems.

As everything in life then has a frequency, deep sleep and healing have a frequency as well. Start your experiment at YouTube with various frequency music videos. These videos can play for 8 or 9 hours, in the background, before you sleep or all the way through your sleep, while prompting you subconsciously to relax, heal and regenerate. Here's a nine-hour YouTube frequency video to try out. And of course, it's free. https://bit.ly/2jWrV4p. By the way, there are hundreds of other frequency videos on hundreds of topics too, from sleep to public speaking, foreign language improvement, and even job interview success while you sleep. Take a little time and try this out. It's a whole new world out there folks.

Stay Hydrated to Ward off Dehydration

You may be sick of people saying "drink more water", but the truth is most people are walking around dehydrated. It's sad, because in a developed country there is no reason for people to be dehydrated and dehydration can cause so many illnesses and lead to exhaustion. You can get very sick, all because you aren't drinking enough water.

Know How Much to Drink

As mentioned before, most people need to drink the equivalent of half their body weight in ounces. Your body is about 65-75% water. It needs water to function properly at every level. So, if you are a 150-pound woman, drink a minimum of 75 ounces of water every day faithfully. This is just a minimum level but you should also go by your thirst level. Start with this amount, and if you're still thirsty, drink more. But, drink this much water each day and begin to feel better. Coffee and soda drinks don't count in this water equation either, and actually work against your water intake. Eliminating sugary drinks from your diet is a great health strategy because of the "empty calories" they have, but also because they work against your body's cell development, tend to break down calcium and bones in the body and cause gastric issues in the gut. See Amazon for a good book on the subject. **Leaky Gut...The Path to Optimal Health.**

Don't guzzle your water. It's not good for you to drink too much water too fast. If you're letting yourself get so thirsty that you're downing a 32-ounce bottle of water in 2 minutes that is not a good idea. It can be dangerous to drink too much water too fast. Instead, try to give yourself water in smaller amounts all throughout the day.

Eat Hydrating Foods

Lots of food is very hydrating, especially raw fruit and vegetables. While you shouldn't drink your food, eating a juicy apple, a slice of watermelon and other fruit is very helpful for getting more hydrated. When you have a choice between something dry and something full of water, choose the thing that is full of water.

Use a Humidifier

While this is not putting water inside your body, it can still help. If you live in a dry climate, are going through a drought, or it's just winter, consider getting a cold air humidifier to keep on at least in your bedroom while you sleep. This will help your body stay more hydrated and keep your sinus passages healthy.

Dehydration can make you very tired and sap you of energy. It can also make you sick. Not drinking enough water can cause chronic headaches, dry skin, dry eyes, and kidney problems. It can also make you disoriented, forgetful, and sap you of energy. When something is as simple as drinking more water to boost your energy, you should do it.

What's more, most of the time drinking water right out of the tap is safe, so there is no reason to use bottled water or any type of special water. It makes it one of the least expensive beauty treatments ever. Take the 30-day water challenge. Try drinking your minimum amount of water for 30 days. Take a before picture, then take an after picture. You're going to be surprised that you look younger and have lost weight too. Plus, you will have a lot more energy to do even more each day.

One thing that helps you be more energetic during the day is a good night's rest. But, most of us do things to make it hard for ourselves to get enough sleep. You can make it better by making your bedroom a sleeping environment.

Make Your Bedroom a Fortress of Comfort

Sleeping is an important part of being more energetic each day. Sadly, most of us no longer have a real bedroom. Instead, we have computers, TVs, and of course, we carry our mobile devices everywhere. We eat in bed, watch TV in bed, talk on the phone in bed, debate on social media in bed – and all that activity makes it much harder to get to get a good night's sleep.

Instead, to have more energy each day and get a really good night's rest, consider making your bedroom into a fortress of comfort designed especially for sleeping. Not always easy in today's world, but you have to make rest and recovery a priority.

* **Minimize** – The less clutter you have in your home, the easier it is going to be to relax and sleep. This is especially true of your bedroom. Set up your bedroom so that everything has a home, and everything is neat. You don't want a lot of clutter on top of furniture to distract you. Keep only what you want and need in your bedroom.

* **Humidify** – Dry air, especially winter air, can cause disturbances during your sleep. Get a cold air humidifier to turn on each night. The ideal air humidity for sleeping should be about 45 percent. Lower risks dry sinus cavities and higher can trigger mold, bacteria, and dust mite issues.

* **Keep It Cool** – The ideal temperature for sleeping is between 60 and 68 degrees Fahrenheit. That might seem cold, but with the right PJs and the right sheets and blankets you should be very comfortable and fall asleep fast. It's the cool face, warm body approach. If it's too warm in the house, you'll have a tendency to

kick off the covers and then lay on them instead of under them. Try this technique for a few nights and see if it doesn't change your sleep pattern.

* **Get a Good Mattress** – Many people skimp on mattresses, but a mattress is one of the most important investments in your health that you can make. You want one that is neither too hard nor too soft, made from natural fibers that support your body to help maintain spine alignment. Some folks swear by sleep number beds that are air filled chambers, and others like foam or pillow top mattresses. Whatever your choice in beds is, get a good one. Test drive the latest beds and select one that serves you best. Remember, you'll spend 6-10 hours a day in bed, so your sleep and health begins with a good night's rest.

* **Spring for the Best Sheets** – Don't be cheap about sheets. You only need two sets so that you can wash your sheets weekly and switch off. Buy at least 400-800 thread count and 100% cotton sheets. Make sure that they fit your bed correctly. Light colors like white are easier to keep clean and stay cooler. Quality sheets and pillowcases always pays off with a restful

sleep. Change weekly or more often as needed. The feeling of clean sheets is very restful.

* **Get the Right Pillows** – The other aspect of sleeping is your pillow. A pillow should support your head so that your spine stays in alignment and so that your head isn't bent or raised higher than it would be naturally lying on your shoulder. Some folks prefer water pillows that conform to neck and shoulders, and still others use foam or fill. Whatever you choose, select a good pillow. Tossing and turning and "fighting your pillow" every night is not restful at all. Make the investment. Get a great pillow that insures your continuous relaxation.

* **Use Layers** – To keep your temperature comfortable, use layers. Sheets, a couple of blankets, and a light comforter is the best in winter weather. You can then remove layers as needed or add them back if you get too cold. Summer's in some hot and humid parts of the country, you'll probably sleep with a sheet and a single blanket. That's okay. Adjust to your sleep patterns consciously.

* **Outlaw Electronics** – Don't let any electronics cross the threshold of your room. Keep TVs out, phones out, and your mobile devices out. The only exception is if you're on call for some type of emergency. Otherwise, understand that the best help you can offer anyone is a good night's sleep so that you're well rested each day.

Good sleep will make you more energized throughout the day. Go to bed and get up at the same time each night and morning.

Ensure Your Nutrition Needs Are Met

Out of all the energy-zapping things you can do, eating wrong and not paying attention to your nutritional needs are two of the most overlooked problem areas. Whether you're exhausted, anxious, suffer from insomnia or just don't feel great, look at your nutrition plan as a first step to getting your energy back. Supplementation is vital to get the appropriate nutrients your body needs.

Take a Blood Test

Ask your doctor for a complete blood work-up to test all your vitamin and hormone levels. You could be short on vitamin B12 or D3. You may also have anemia, which is a shortage of iron. You may even have a thyroid condition causing you to be tired all the time. All of these can easily be fixed if you follow through. Seek out those on your medical team that can help and direct you.

Eat Healthy, Eat Clean

Whether you eat a high-carb, plant-based, or low-carb diet, they teach the same thing. Stop eating processed food. Get rid of anything that is processed including sugar, bread, sugary snacks and so forth. If it's not grown out of the ground, or organic, antibiotic free, or grass fed, don't buy it. Then just eat half your calories in vegetables, about a fourth in fruit, and fill the rest with fat and protein. It's that easy, regardless of which diet you're on. If you're eating only high nutrient food, you'll be able to feel good fast.

Avoid Fast Food

Don't go through a drive-thru. Have you heard the expression before..."that nothing ever good, comes through a drive-thru window?" If you go to any restaurants, try to eat a great salad and grilled meat. At home, it's quick to cook this type of food. A fast dinner is to bake sweet potato in the microwave, steam some veggies, and heat up some beans. If you want meat, simply put it in the oven for about thirty minutes. Keeping it simple works best. Weekly and even monthly meal planning, saves you time, money and the daily frustration of "what's for dinner tonight?" from family members. If everyone knows the meal plan, you can regulate diets easier and aid in sleep that night too.

Make a Plan, Work Your Plan

The best thing to do is plan everything. Before you walk into a grocery store, know what you're going to buy and why. Know what nutrients you're trying to fulfill before you buy or eat anything. Try your best to avoid your cravings while you shop. If you are eating something for flavor only, then you may be making a crucial health mistake. It's okay to eat things that taste good, but know why you're eating them. Having a menu plan really helps.

Finally, make sure you eat at the right time. Recent studies have shown that if weight loss is a concern for you, then eating only from 12-8pm will keep you burning calories during your day. "Intermittent Fasting" is becoming a lifestyle change that yields real promise as the weight loss is real. One of the keys to intermittent fasting though is to not eat after 8pm, so the body can digest and recover before bedtime. Try it. You're literally fasting for 16 hours while your body is burning calories constantly. Share your results on my FaceBook page. **Optimal Health**. I'd love to read your stories and testimonials.

For many of us however, continue to eat something for breakfast, lunch, and dinner, and if you're still hungry, sometimes you can eat a healthy snack or two a day. Don't let your hunger dictate to you. You plan for it. Remember, a handful of almonds is a snack. One apple is a snack. You don't have to be stuffed every time you eat. Try to eat at least 2-3 hours before you go to bed so that you can sleep better without having to worry about digestion.

There's an insomnia and anxiety link in children and teens that is often overlooked by parents and therapists. I've included a bonus chapter below with suggestions on how to best help children maximize their sleep and rest periods as well.

CONCLUSION

As you have learned in this book, sleep is just as important as healthy eating and exercise. It is a complex process consisting of stages that pass from Non-REM to REM. Your brain is active at all these stages, and it is responsible for restoring your energy, decreasing your susceptibility to infections and diseases, in helping your body's tissues repair themselves and grow, and in consolidating new memories and learning.

Unfortunately, many people are not getting the quality sleep that their bodies require. Medical conditions –

physical or psychological – can sometimes be the cause. Fortunately, things can be done to improve your sleep, even if you have a medical condition.

However, not all sleep problems are caused by medical issues. Many are the result of poor sleep hygiene and lifestyle choices, such as the use of technology and artificial lighting before bedtime. By making changes in your environment - via lighting and temperature control, as examples – your sleep can improve significantly.

By understanding the stages of sleep, and applying the tips in this book, you can begin to experience a better sleep from now on. As previously mentioned, quantity is not the only aspect of good sleep. Quality is key.

So what are you waiting for? Begin by putting these tips into action as early as tonight, and see how your sleep improves! And speaking of tips, here's a few more that can kick-start your new sleeping regimen.

Here in the next chapter, are 11 Energizing Tips and Hacks to get you back on track with your sleep regimen. Enjoy.

ZZZ's

BONUS

The Insomnia & Anxiety Link in Children & Teens and What Parents Need To Do To Help

"Sleep Solves Almost Everything. Dear Bed, I Love You.

Good night! ~Bob Armstrong

Introduction

If you have difficulty falling asleep, staying asleep, or waking up early in the morning, you may be suffering from insomnia. It is not enough to close your eyes, and simply count sheep and hope you will enter the world of slumber. Most people, of ALL ages, have occasional insomnia at some point in their lives, experiencing it due to changes in sleep schedules (as during travel and vacations) or stressful circumstances, for example.

However, when it starts happening frequently and becomes long term, it can really cause problems in your day to day functioning. You may feel sleepy putting you and others at increased risk of injury if you drive a vehicle or operate machinery. You may also have trouble concentrating, and experience problems with your memory. When you are not getting enough sleep due to insomnia, little stressors can feel like huge stressors, and your coping skills deteriorate. As a result, your relationships with your family, friends, and/or co-workers can suffer as well.

To complicate matters, people with insomnia often also have anxiety or an anxiety disorder. Further complicating things, if you have both anxiety and depression, your insomnia is often worse.

So why does anxiety and insomnia often co-exist in individuals?

There are two ways to look at this. Insomnia can cause the anxiety, OR anxiety can cause the insomnia. It's common for them to exist together however.

First, let's discuss how insomnia can cause the anxiety. If you are having trouble sleeping, this may lead to anxiety about a number of different things. You might start worrying about how you will function the next day on so little sleep, and how you will ever make it through the entire day. As you think about this and watch the numbers on the clock slowly advance, you become more anxious, making it even more difficult to fall asleep.

On the other hand, when your anxiety is causing the insomnia, your anxiety makes it difficult to shut off thoughts in your head. You may be feeling worried or fearful about perceived or real issues. An example that a new parent may experience is that of having a newborn baby who sleeps very poorly at night. It may feel like every time you start to fall asleep, that the baby wakes up. In someone prone to anxiety, this may translate into anxious thoughts (i.e. "The baby is going to wake up just as I start to fall asleep.") when you go to bed, resulting in the inability to fall asleep. In the case of a child with anxiety that results in insomnia, the anxiety may revolve around the fear of the dark or being alone away from his parents.

Because anxiety and insomnia are so prevalent in children and teens today, it is a topic worthy of discussion on its own.

Is insomnia in children and teens similar to adults?

Yes, children can have insomnia as well. In fact, a poll done by the National Sleep Foundation found that more than two out of three children ten years old and under have had a sleep issue of some sort.

Insomnia may last for only a few days (due to sickness), or it can become more frequent and long-term. Sometimes this can be indicative of anxiety, depression, or other medical problems, so you should always make sure to have your child evaluated by their pediatrician.

Obviously, children and teens may have different reasons for their insomnia when compared to adults. For example, children may be scared of the monsters they think exist in their closets or under their beds. Teens may be stressed by exams or bullying going on at school. In many cases, there is a component of anxiety that coexists with the insomnia. That is why it is important to try to get to the **root cause** of the insomnia whenever possible. In some cases, there is no particular reason for the insomnia, however.

The signs and symptoms of insomnia in children and teens can include:

- Sleepiness during the day

- Poor performance in school

- Irritability

- Anxiety

- Decreased focus and concentration

- Mood swings

- Being worried about things

- Hyperactivity

- Forgetfulness and decreased memory for things

- Increased behavioral issues such as fighting and not getting along with others

- Increased impulsiveness

Because children and teens with insomnia have been found to have increased risk for anxiety disorders and depression, it is important to recognize the signs and symptoms of insomnia in your children and teens so that you can help ensure they get the sleep they need. Here are some ways to help a child or teen with insomnia.

- **Try to determine the cause of the insomnia first**

For example, if you learn that your child is stressed by trying to keep up with school and homework as well as out-of-school extracurricular activities, you will need to address this before the insomnia can go away. This can be quite a common stressor for children and teens, as they tend to be overscheduled.

- **Once you determine the cause, try to eliminate the stressor**

In the example above, if the problem is the child feeling stressed by an overly busy schedule, you will need to make adjustments to the schedule. It may involve talking to the teacher, and setting realistic expectations for homework. Perhaps you will learn that your child is not using his time effectively at school and home, and he therefore needs more guidance on how to do this.

Many children and teens are poor managers of their time, and they will need your help in this area. To do this, you may need to set limits on use of technology such as video games, for example. It may also be helpful to sit down and help your child determine how to prioritize tasks.

- **Establish and follow a bedtime routine**

Just like younger children do well with a set routine every night, so do older children (teens and even adults). It gets your mind and body prepared for sleep. When you have a set routine, it also keeps things predictable and allows you to manage your time better.

You need to teach children and teens that they need time to unwind and relax before actually going to sleep. This means no television, video games, social media, and so forth for one to two hours before going to bed. These bright devices can also interfere with melatonin production in your body, which helps tell your body that it is time to go to sleep.

Instead, teach them that they can do something relaxing such as reading a book before turning off the light, if they are old enough. Invest in special light bulbs that do not emit blue light. Red light bulbs are also an option, and you can find them online. For younger children, you can set up a specific routine of having a bedtime snack, then teeth brushing, you read them a book, and then tuck them into bed with a hug and kiss. It may also help to provide your child with a back rub or some extra cuddling time. You just have to determine what works best for your own children.

- **Limit your child's or teen's access to the news**

Unfortunately, the news media portrays a lot of violent and terrible things happening in the world – from terrorist activities to inclement weather such as tornadoes and floods. For an already-anxious child, this can severely contribute to insomnia.

- **Do not discuss anxiety-provoking or stressful situations before bedtime**

Before your child goes to bed, it is not the time to discuss your disappointment in your child's grades or that he forgot to do his chores again.

- **Teach your older child stress manage-ment and anxiety-reducing techniques**

Children with insomnia can benefit from many of the same stress and anxiety reduction techniques that adults use – progressive muscle relaxation, visual imagery, yoga, prayer and deep diaphragmatic breathing.

Learning these methods and using them before bed, can help treat insomnia as they can turn on the relaxed, parasympathetic part of your nervous system.

- **Teach and use good sleep hygiene methods**

These methods include waking up and going to bed at the same time, avoiding napping, and avoiding caffeinated beverages and foods six hours before bedtime.

Ensure the bed is only used for sleep, and that it is not the place where the child watches television or does other activities during the day.

In addition, do not exercise two hours before bedtime. However, do keep in mind that exercise is important in helping with quality sleep so do ensure you do promote exercise. The best kinds of activities can be those where you spend time with your child going for a walk, riding a bike, or going to the park.

Also teach your older child that instead of tossing and turning for too long, it is better to get out of bed, put a light on low (preferably a red light bulb), and do something quiet such as reading for 15 minutes, and then go back to bed and attempt to sleep. If sleep does not occur soon after returning to bed, then he can get up again, and repeat the process until sleep finally does come.

• **Set up the bedroom for rest and relaxation**

This means sleeping in a room that is not overly hot. It is recommended that you keep the room between 68 and 70 degrees Fahrenheit (20 – 21 degrees Celsius). It really does depend on the age of the child and if/what types of pajamas the child wears to bed.

Have drapes in place to keep the room dark during sleeping, but you can have a small unobtrusive nightlight (with a red light bulb) in a corner of the room, if necessary to lessen anxiety. If your child tends to stare at the alarm clock numbers, then it is best to turn it around to make sure that it is not able to be viewed.

• **Remove technology devices from the bedroom**

In the age of electronics, video games, TV and visual entertainment stimulus, it's difficult to remove everything from your bedroom. But removing temptation to check the time, text messages, emails, or social media for the latest updates can reduce anxiety and stress too.

Keep in mind, that anxiety stressors, especially if there is anything unsettling that your child reads or views just before bedtime makes it difficult to go to sleep. The blue light emitted from these devices also suppresses melatonin – the sleep hormone – thereby delaying sleep further.

In children with anxiety, removal of the devices during the day can also be helpful. Initially, it may cause more anxiety due to the fear of not being accessible by others and no longer "being in the loop" at all times. This FOMO, or Fear of Missing Out, can be its own anxiety provoking issue. However, you can teach your children that being "on call" all the time or knowing every little thing about other people's lives (through social media), can cause them more anxiety and unneeded stress which further contributes to their sleep problems.

- **Spend extra time with your children and teens**

When you spend time talking and doing fun things together (i.e. family board game night, movies, taekwondo together, etc.), your children will feel closer to you, trust you more, and will open up to you more fully. This gives you the opportunity to get a better idea of what they are experiencing in their lives, and how it may be contributing to their insomnia and anxiety. Many times, you can also help reduce the insomnia by helping them deal with or solve the problems that they are facing. You have to remember that children and teens do not have the life experience and knowledge of how to deal with situations like you do. By simply providing them with this guidance and teaching, you can help reduce the anxiety too. Encourage communication and trust every day in your relationship with your children.

In addition, you want to remember that you want to teach them methods of how they can deal with stressors when you are not around. You may want to do some role playing to give them the confidence to deal with situations that arise when you cannot be present. Practice role-playing perhaps, on the drive to school?

- **Consult a physician or naturopathic doctor**

Sometimes, more help is needed. Consider consulting a member of your "health team" also. Medications are not generally prescribed for children with insomnia. However, alternative treatment options may include cognitive-behavioral therapy. The physician or pediatrician can make a referral to a therapist or psychologist trained in this area.

A naturopathic doctor may also be able to provide natural suggestions for improving sleep too.

In any case, it is always important for the healthcare professional to try to determine if there is a physical or psychological cause to your child's insomnia.

Just the Beginning

Insomnia is a problem for adults, children, and teens and almost all suffer from it at various times in their lives. Anxiety often co-exists in individuals with insomnia, and so it becomes important to identify the source of the anxiety if insomnia is to be treated successfully. There are many methods that can be used to help a child with insomnia, which have been outlined above.

Try tracking your sleep over the next 30-60 days. By measuring what insomnia triggers you can eliminate, you can better prepare and plan for your good night's sleep. Below, in the resource section, are some "free sleep journals and diaries" in Adobe .pdf format so you can download and save them. But use them. There are several to choose from. These should help you to track your sleep cycles effectively. Let's face it, the more you know about your sleep patterns, the better health you will enjoy for the rest of your life. It's worth the few minutes each day to fill-in the blanks. I've also included for you additional research and sleep studies. Please take a little time and review them too.

For you, a restful and rejuvenating sleep can begin today with the information here and your commitment to make a few small lifestyle changes. I know you can do it. Millions have gone on before you and are now enjoying the benefits of restful and replenishing sleep. You've got this.

Finally, for most of us, know that there's a desire to do just a little more at the end of every day. To push ourselves a little further. And while that sounds noble and good, I also believe that our sleep, exercise and diet are just as important as any goal we may have. So stop and consider your health first and most important.

So, the first step to improving our sleep, exercise and diet is to make them a top priority in our life. So achieving one more to-do list item, should be no substitute for taking the best care of your body (and your health) today. As Jim Rohn once stated, "take care of your body, it's the only place you have to live."

Thank you for taking the time to read and explore how amazing sleep is and its value to your health. Please leave a positive comment with Amazon if you have found some value in these pages. It really helps. Thank you. For my other books in the Optimal Health Series, please check out my author page at **Bob Armstrong**.

RESOURCES

Free Sleep Journals:

https://thebettersleepproject.com/sleep-diary/

http://yoursleep.aasmnet.org/pdf/sleepdiary.pdf

https://www.nhs.uk/Livewell/insomnia/Documents/sleepdiary.pdf

http://www.healthysleep.med.harvard.edu/file/19

www.pa-foundation.org/wp-content/uploads/NSF-Sleep-Diary.pdf

Sleep Diary for Kids

www.sleepforkids.org/pdf/SleepDiary.pdf

Sleep Studies & Tests

https://www.ncbi.nlm.nih.gov/pubmed/20669438

https://www.aastweb.org/blog/5-types-of-sleep-study-tests-and-when-to-use-them (5 different tests)

https://my.clevelandclinic.org/health/articles/12131-sleep-studies

https://www.sleepdr.com/the-sleep-blog/10-of-the-most-important-things-you-need-to-know-about-sleep/

https://www.huffingtonpost.com/entry/uk-sleep-report-calls-for-national-sleep-strategy_us_56fda1fde4b0daf53aef4dd9

https://www.hopkinsmedicine.org/health/healthy-sleep/sleep-science/the-future-of-sleep-studies

Sleep Statistics

http://www.sleepmedsite.com/page/sb/sleep_disorders/sleep_statistics

From the **Optimal Business Series** of books, Bob has also written a very timely business book for Amazon Kindle & Paperback readers...

1001 Business Ideas

Finding the Right Business to Fuel Your Passion and Create Your Perfect Lifestyle

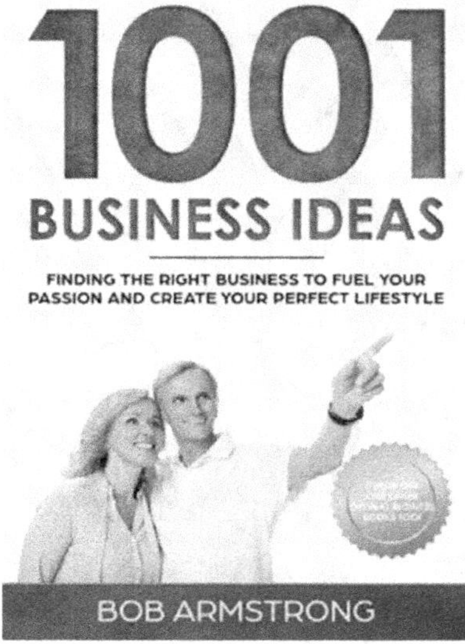

If you or someone you know is looking to start a new business and need a 1001 ideas...this is it!

Thank you so much. ~Bob Armstrong

ZZZ's